Daoist

Body

Cultivation

Traditional Models
and
Contemporary Practices

edited
by
Livia Kohn

Three Pines Press
P.O. Box 207
Magdalena, NM 87825
www.threepinespress.com

9   8 7 6 5 4 3 2 1

Printed in the United States of America
⊗ This edition is printed on acid-free paper that meets
the American National Standard Institute Z39.48 Standard.
Distributed in the United States by Three Pines Press.

Cover Art: "The Six Healing Sounds," by Juan Li. Used with permission, Mantak Chia, http://universal-tao.com.

Library of Congress Cataloging-in-Publication Data

Daoist body cultivation: traditional models and contemporary practices / edited by Livia Kohn.

p. cm.
Includes bibliographical references and index.
ISBN   1-931483-05-1   (alk. paper)
    1.   Health-Religious aspects—Taoism. 2. Hygiene, Taoist.
    2.   I. Kohn, Livia, 1956-
    RA 776.5.D327   2006
    613.2—dc22
    2005037747

Contents

Illustrations

Introduction

Many religious traditions encourage the practice of cultivation. They support their members in developing qualities that are seen as ideal, perfect, or desirable within the context of their beliefs, qualities that make their followers more like the deity or cosmic principle at their core. Thus, for example, Christians encourage the development of neighborly love, unselfishness, and social services. Buddhists like to see their followers be morally upright, calmly self-possessed, and full of wisdom. In each case, the object of cultivation is closely correlated to the sacred, the central concern, and most divine aspect of the religion, while human life on its ordinary, mundane level is seen as separate and different from this vision. We are by our nature of being human not ideal or perfect. We lack inner peace, mutual love, and divinity. We are not like the deity or the cosmic principle—but we have the spark, the seed, the trace of the divine within us.

Cultivation thus presupposes two basic assumptions. One, that human life and the human condition are divergent from the divine, the ultimate, the perfection. And two, that there is the potential for attaining the perfect state within every human being. The practice of cultivation, then, just like its agricultural counterpart in the mundane world, means to plant the seed, support and nurture it, keep predators and weeds away, allow it to grow, and gradually raise it to full bloom. Eventually the seed will be a completely grown plant, and cultivation will no longer be a separate practice but will become one with life itself. In the religious context, this means that to understand cultivation one should first examine the ideals and goals of the religion in question, then find the nature of the seed and look for the different methods of care and cultivation.

Consistent with the growth metaphor, cultivation means action and forward motion, progress and enhancement. Once begun, it is a continuous process, an ongoing movement of transformation. It requires that one challenges basic assumptions about self and world, becomes a new person with every phase, and is never quite satisfied, done, or finished. There is always the divine ideal looming above. There is always yet another step to take, another area to support, another aspect to work on. The process itself, the journey to the goal, becomes

1

the way of cultivation, and for the dedicated practitioner that is his life.

Just as in planting a field one can rely entirely on oneself or get help from manuals, advisers, and assistants, so cultivation can be undertaken either under one's own steam or with the help of others. The Japanese tradition distinguishes this most clearly in its contrast between Zen and Pure Land, described as *jiriki* 自力 or "self-power" and *tariki* 他力 or "other power," respectively. In other words, to cultivate the religious ideal one can follow a path of self-transformation through virtue, meditation, and self-control or one can deliver oneself into the hands of a deity or divine agent, a bodhisattva-type savior who will give support and guidance and even take matters into his or her powerful hands. Another image sometimes used in the Buddhist context is that of the bicycle versus the bus. Both will take you to the desired destination, but on the bicycle you have to propel yourself forward by your own strength, whereas on the bus you can leave the driving and decision-making to someone else.

It may seem at first glance that biking is a great deal harder than sitting on a bus, but the fact is that human beings have a very difficult time delivering themselves unquestioningly into the hands of another, however much revered, beloved, and trusted. Giving oneself in devotion is just as hard, and for some people may be even harder, than pursuing the mystical path of meditation and self-control.

You may note at this point that we speak of "trusting" and "self-control," both essentially mental actions and psychological attitudes. And indeed, in most traditions the path of cultivation, whichever form it may take, is one of mental transformation. More than anything, it requires a change in attitude and awareness, a development of qualities such as compassion, neighborly love, calmness, and detachment—all essentially unphysical, not of the body. Bodies tend to be on the sidelines of cultivation, at best left to their own devices, at worst maligned and mistreated. All too often the basic human nature of greediness and egotism is understood to be rooted in the fact that we have bodies and that these bodies have needs that have to be satisfied. As Bertold Brecht, the famous German dramatist, says in his *Three Penny Opera*: "Erst kommt das Fressen, dann kommt die Moral!" or "Food first, ethics later." Yes, it is very hard to be good if you are poor, hungry, dirty, and disheveled. And all too often the residents of monasteries, the cultivation sites *par excellence*, are well fed, well clothed, well kept, and in general freed from bodily worries.

But there is another alternative to taking the body out of the cultivation equation. That is, one can make the body the basis, the root, the foundation of the cultivation process, anchor oneself in physicality and transform the very nature of bodily existence as part of the divine undertaking. This is the route the Daoist tradition has chosen—a unique route that has yet to find its match among other religions and that has, with physicality becoming more relevant these days, a great appeal to modern Western seekers. Would not it be nice, really, to enjoy the body and be a good person, both at the same time? Would it not be nice to be able to enjoy all sorts of treats and pleasures while also moving forward on the path to divine existence?

There is great appeal in this vision, and the Chinese tradition, life-affirming and world-loving from the beginning, has explored it extensively. Their solution to the problem of having a body and wanting to be divine is something called *qi* 氣.

Qi and the Five Phases

Qi is the foundational energy of the universe, the basic stuff of the Dao, the life force in the human body, and the basis of all physical vitality. Tangible in the sensations and pulses, visible as vapor and breath, audible in sighs and sounds, it is what we are as physical, embodied beings. Yet it is also the material energy of Dao, the underlying force of the greater universe, the power that makes things happen in the cosmos. There is only one *qi*, just as there is only one Dao, and through it people and the cosmos are one. We are by way of being bodies already part of the divine, the ultimate, the creation. All we have to do is realize this fact and behave accordingly.

That is to say, not all is well by just being *qi*. *Qi* appears on different levels and in different modes. At our core, in our deepest being, there are the cosmic forms of primordial and prenatal *qi*, i.e., *qi* that is part of the creative substratum of the universe and the true, perfect *qi* we receive from our parents. At the periphery, in our lives and day-to-day expression, there is postnatal or earthly *qi*. All three have to work together smoothly and with ease for health and harmony to be achieved.

Health, then, is not just the absence of symptoms and ailments. It is the presence of a strong vital energy and a smooth, harmonious, and active flow of *qi*. This is known as the state of *zhengqi* 正氣 or "proper *qi*," also translated as "upright *qi*." The ideal is to have *qi* flow freely, creating harmony in the body and a balanced state of being in the person. This personal health is further matched by health in nature, defined as regular weather patterns and the absence of disasters. It is also present as health in society in the peaceful coexistence among families, clans, villages, and states. This harmony on all levels, the cosmic presence of a steady and pleasant flow of *qi*, is what the Chinese call the state of Great Peace (*taiping* 太平), a state venerated by all different religious, philosophical, and political schools in traditional China.

The opposite of health, what other traditions would describe as turning away from the divine and giving in to bodily urges, in China is *xieqi* 邪氣 or "wayward *qi*," also called deviant *qi*, pathogenic *qi*, heteropathic *qi*, or evil *qi*. In a condition of *xieqi*, humans have lost their harmonious relation to the cosmos, the *qi* field has fallen out of balance, and people's *qi* no longer supports the dynamic forces of change. Whereas proper *qi* moves in a smooth, steady rhythm and effects daily renewal, helping health and long life, wayward *qi* is disorderly and dysfunctional and creates change that violates the normal order. When it becomes dominant, the *qi*-flow can turn upon itself and deplete the body's resources. The individual loses his or her connection to the universe, no longer operates as part of a greater system, and is increasingly out of tune with the basic life force.

This in due course results in irritation: mental irritation that appears as negative emotions and physical irritation that shows up as bodily discomforts and eventually leads to disease. People have the ability to feel the quality of their *qi* within their bodies. They also have the power to regulate its flow, and they have the strength to control its intake and output. The same applies to the levels of nature and society. In nature, wayward *qi* means the occurrence of unpredictable weather patterns, such as floods, droughts, locust plagues, earthquakes, and the like. In society, it means upheaval in rebellions, revolutions, or acts of terrorism. As in the body, these signs of uneven *qi* flow can be predicted, controlled, and remedied—provided one understands the subtle dynamic of life on all its levels.

This fundamental understanding of the body and the divine is common to all of Chinese culture and finds its best-known expression in Chinese medicine as well as, to a less well-known degree, in Chinese political theory. The Daoist tradition, as the indigenous higher religion of China, has developed it further by linking the body with the natural world and with the country's administration, by populating it with stellar deities, and by defining subtler distinctions and types of energy. On this basis, it has created an intricate, complex system of spiritual cultivation, through which the body is transformed energetically into the subtlest possible potency. Its ultimate goal is to become one with the Dao, to reach a state of mystical union and release of personal ego-identity on this earth and to ascend to the heavens of the gods and immortals after death.

The body in Daoism as a system of *qi* is part and parcel of the natural world.[1] Its every part matches one or the other aspect of nature, so that already the *Huainanzi* 淮南子 (Writings of the Prince of Huainan) of the second century B.C.E. says that "the roundness of the head is an image of Heaven, the squareness of the feet follows the pattern of Earth." Just as the natural world functions according to the four seasons, five phases, nine directions, and 360 days, "human beings have four limbs, five inner organs, nine orifices, and 360 joints." Similarly, the various forces of nature, such as wind, rain, cold, and heat are matched in people's "actions of giving, taking, joy, and anger." Each organ, moreover, has a part to play in the natural inner world: "The gall bladder corresponds to the clouds, the lungs to the breath, the liver to the wind, the kidneys to the rain, and the spleen to the thunder" (ch. 7; see Major 1978).

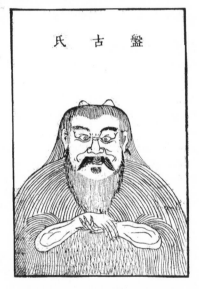

Fig. 1: Pangu, the Creator

A more radical vision of the same idea appears in the Daoist adaptation of the Indian myth of Puruṣa, where the physical body of the deity is transformed into the world (see Lincoln 1975). In China this story is first told about the creator figure Pangu 盤古, it also appears with the defied Laozi as key protagonist (see Fig. 1). The story goes:

> Laozi changed his body. His left eye became the sun and his right eye the moon. His head was Mount Kunlun, his hair the stars. His bones turned into dragons, his flesh into wild

---

[1] The following discussion of the body in Daoism is based on Kohn 1991. Other presentations are found in Homann 1971; Schipper 1978; 1994; Ishida 1989; Andersen 1994; Kroll 1996; Saso 1997; Bumbacher 2001; Despeux 2005.

> beasts, his intestines into snakes. His breast was the ocean,
> his fingers, the five sacred mountains. The hair on his body
> was transformed into grass and trees, his heart into the
> constellation Cassiopeia. Finally, his testicles joined in em-
> brace as the true parents of the universe. (*Xiaodao lun*;
> Kohn 1995, 55)

Here every obvious part of the body—eyes, ears, hair, bones, limbs, intestines—is transformed into an aspect of nature, creating a com-plete and systematic match of the human body and the larger uni-verse.

Under the Han dynasty (206 B.C.E.-220 C.E.), Chinese cosmologists created an even more sophisticated matching of body parts and as-pects of the natural world by classifying the entire universe as well as the body's parts and activities according to yin 陰 and yang 陽 and further subdividing this into the so-called five phases (*wuxing* 五行). That is to say, they took the two forces yin and yang and not only linked them with any number of complementary opposites in the hu-man, natural, and cosmic levels (e.g., low and high, cold and warm, female and male, earth and heaven), but also interpreted them as continuously evolving from one into the other. As yin rises and grows, it reaches its zenith and gives way to yang, which in its turn rises and grows until it reaches its zenith, and so on. They duly identified five phases of yin and yang and associated them with five material objects as their appropriate symbols. The five phases and their symbols are:

minor yang	major yang	yin-yang	minor yin	major yin
wood	fire	earth	metal	water

In the human body, these five phases are present as the five inner organs (*wuzang* 五臟; liver, heart, spleen, lungs, kidneys), which also work together in a constant flow of movement and exchange. They may have names like the organs we know from Western medicine, but they are more than mere organs. They serve as the receptacles and centers of an entire network of *qi*, and any reference made to any of them connotes the entire fabric of functional manifestations related to them. Consequently "liver" is not just the organ as we know it, but includes the working of muscles and sinews and also corresponds to the sense of vision and the eyes (Porkert 1974, 117-23). Beyond the five phases, the five inner organs are further associated with planets, geographical directions, colors, seasons, digestive organs, emotions, senses, and spiritual forces. This set of correspondences provides an intricate system that thoroughly mixes the cosmic with the physical and directly reflects the fundamental worldview of the body and universe being one through *qi*. Its main components are:

> *liver*: wood, east, green, spring, gallbladder, anger, eyes, spirit soul
> *heart*: fire, south, red, summer, small intestine, agitation, tongue, spirit
> *spleen*: earth, center, yellow, late summer, stomach, worry, lips, will
> *lungs*: metal, west, white, fall, large int., sadness, nose, material soul
> *kidneys*: water, north, black, winter, bladder, fear, ears, essence

As centers of a network of *qi* both on the physical and cosmic levels, the five organs are also the focal points of the so-called meridians or conduits of *qi* that run along the arms and legs to and from the extremities and connect the center of the body to its periphery. They are analogous to the earth arteries in the natural world, described and analyzed by Fengshui specialists and responsible for the auspicious or unlucky placement of houses and graves. In either case, *qi* needs to flow freely—a process helped by the correct construction of manmade structures as much as by physical cultivation methods.

One way of envisioning the correct management of the body's organs and inner resources is through the metaphor of an administrative system. This vision appears first in the medical classics, such as the *Huangdi neijing suwen* 黃帝內經素問 (The Yellow Emperor's Inner Classic, Simple Questions). It says:

> The heart is the residence of the ruler: spirit and clarity originate here. The lungs are the residence of the high ministers of state: order and division originate here. The liver is the residence of the strategists: planning and organization originate here. The gall is residence of the judges: judgments and decisions originate here.
>
> The center of the breast is the residence of a special taskforce: joy and pleasure originate here. The stomach is the residence of the granary administration: the various kinds of taste originate here. The large intestine is the residence of the teachers of the Dao: development and transformations originate here. . . . The kidneys are the residence of the business men: activity and care originate here (3.1ab).

Understanding the body in this way, one can give special attention to parts that are underdeveloped with the ultimate goal of having all the different aspects work in complete harmony and with maximum efficiency of *qi*-flow. This state, then, is not only essential for physical health but also provides mental ease and allows a subtler sense of going along with the larger patterns of the world. The alchemist Ge Hong 葛洪 accordingly says in his *Baopuzi* 抱朴子 (Book of the Master Who Embraces Simplicity, DZ1185;[2] trl. Ware 1966) of the early fourth century:

> The body of an individual can be pictured as a state. The diaphragm may be compared with the palace; the arms and legs, with the suburbs and frontiers. The bones and joints are like the officials; the inner gods are like the sovereign; the blood is like the ministers of state; the *qi* is like the population.

> Therefore, anyone able to regulate his own body can regulate a state. To take good care of the population is the best way to make your state secure; by the same token, to nurture the *qi* is the way to keep the body whole, for when the population scatters, a state goes to ruin; when the *qi* is exhausted, the body dies. (18.4b)

Just as a good ruler and administrator has to make sure the people are secure and can do their work without impediment, a practitioner of Daoist cultivation needs to tend most urgently to his or her *qi*, ensuring that it is present in adequate quantities, flows smoothly and harmoniously, and does not enter or leave the body improperly. The idea that *qi* is like the population of a state goes well with the concept that the inner organs are its ministries while the joints are its officials. They all have an important part to play, but the central focus of cultivation practice is *qi*, and all other parts are nurtured only through the *qi* and for the *qi*.

Divine Dimensions

An expanded vision of the body as the natural world appears in the medieval Daoist school of Highest Clarity (Shangqing 上清). According to this, the human body is not only a combination of natural patterns and energies but also an inner sphere containing supernatural landscapes and divine beings. The body is a complete world with mountains and rivers, a divine and cosmic realm, a paradise and residence of the gods.

---

[2] Texts in the Daoist canon and its supplements, throughout this volume, are numbered according to Komjathy 2002; Schipper and Verellen 2004.

This understanding appears first in the *Huangting jing* 黃庭經 (Yellow Court Scripture), a visualization manual from the fourth century C.E. In a more recent visual depiction, it is found in the *Neijing tu* 內經圖 (Chart of Interior Passages). Here the celestial headquarters within are located in the head and match the immortals' paradise of Mount Kunlun. It is depicted as a large, luscious mountain surrounded by a wide lake and covered with splendid palaces and wondrous orchards (see Fig. 2: *Neijing tu*).

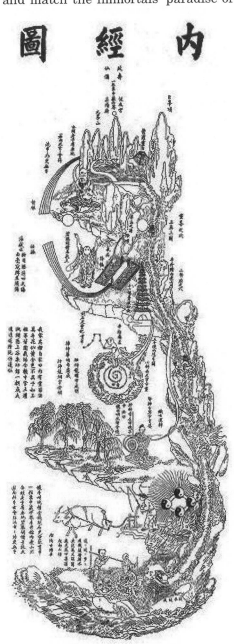

Between the eyes, which are the sun and the moon, one can move inside to the Hall of Light, one of nine palaces in the head. Best reached by passing through the deep, dark valley of the nose, it is guarded by the two high towers of the ears. To attain entry one has to perform the physical/ritual exercise of "beating the heavenly drum": with both palms covering the ears, snap the index and middle fingers to drum against the back of the skull.

Underneath the valley of the nose is a small lake, i.e., the mouth. This regulates the water level of the upper lake in the head and raises or lowers it as necessary. Crossing the mouth-lake over its bridge (tongue) and moving further down, one reaches the twelve-storied tower of the throat, then comes to the Scarlet Palace (heart), the Yellow Court (spleen), the Imperial Granary (stomach),

the Purple Chamber (gall), and various other starry palaces trans-
posed into the body's depth. Going ever deeper, another cosmic region
is reached, with another sun and moon (kidneys). Beneath them, the
Ocean of *Qi* extends with another Mount Kunlun in its midst. Various
divine beings, moreover, reside in the body, creating vitality and providing spiritual resources.

The Daoist vision of the body as a network of celestial passageways
and starry palaces closely overlaps with the medical understanding of
the body as consisting of various aspects of *qi* and the phase-
energetics of the five organs and six viscera. Many acupuncture
points have Daoist connotations, and Chinese healing practices and
physical longevity exercises are at the root of Daoist practice. Without
losing any aspect of the medical dynamics, the Daoist vision provides
a more cosmic and spiritual dimension of the same basic understanding, allowing adepts to move beyond mundane existence toward a
greater, more spiritual realm, reaching out for the gods in the stars
and thereby for the Dao at the center.

While physical practices prepare the body for the higher stages, to
reach the ultimate goal adepts engage in more advanced techniques
of meditation and visualization. One rather well known method is the
interior fixation of the three major Daoist gods in charge of the human body: the Female One, the Male One, and the Great One. They
reside in the upper, middle, and lower energy centers of the body,
commonly known as the cinnabar or elixir fields (*dantian* 丹田) located in the center of the head, solar plexus, and lower abdomen. The
gods are essentially astral divinities, born directly from the primordial energy of the universe in the Northern Dipper, the central con-
stellation of the sky (see Robinet 1993).

Adepts visualize the Three Ones as manifestations of three kinds of
cosmic primordial *qi* in the three elixir fields. They in turn govern the
twenty-four fundamental powers of the human body which correspond to the twenty-four energies of the year and the twenty-four
constellations in the sky. The exact procedure of the meditation varies according to season, but if at all possible should be performed at
the solstices and the equinoxes.

To prepare for the practice, adepts have to purify themselves by bathing and fasting. They enter the meditation chamber at midnight, the
hour of rising yang. Then they light incense, and click their teeth
thirty times. Facing east, they close their eyes and visualize the
Northern Dipper slowly descending toward them until it rests right

above their heads with the handle pointing straight east. This preliminary measure serves to protect adepts from evil influences during the practice.

Then they start with the Upper One. They visualize a ball of red energy in the Niwan Palace, the upper elixir field in the center of the head. Within this ball of energy, a red sun about nine inches in radius will appear. Its brilliance envelops practitioners to such a degree that they enter a state of utter oblivion. As soon as they have reached this state, the god Red Child becomes visible. The ruler of the Niwan Palace, he holds a talisman of the white tiger, the sacred animal of the west. He is accompanied by an attendant, the god of the subtle essences of the teeth, the tongue, and the skull, who holds a sacred scripture in his hands.

The Middle and Lower Ones are similarly imagined as residing in the other elixir fields, the Scarlet Palace of the heart and the Ocean of *Qi* in the abdomen and are accompanied by assistants who govern the five inner organs as well as the extremities, senses, and fluids of the body. Through visualization, adepts keep them securely in the body and over time learn to communicate with them, resulting in the attainment of yet higher stages in which adepts transpose the visualized gods back to their true realm in the stars and paradises and themselves take flight to visit those extraterrestrial realms—dimensions that will be their true home once their limited existence on this earth has come to an end (see Robinet 1993).

Reorienting the body to be the container of heavenly palaces and deities, to be in fact a cosmos in itself, adepts attain oneness in body and spirit with the cosmic dimensions of the universe. As all parts of the body are transformed into divine entities and firmly guarded by their responsible gods, the very physicality of the adept turns into a cosmic network and becomes the celestial realm in which the gods reside. Visualizing and feeling the gods within the bodily self, the Daoist becomes a more cosmic being, transforming but not relinquishing his physical, embodied nature.

Levels of Qi

This physical nature, however, at the higher stages of oneness with gods and cosmic powers, is not the same gross material we experience in ordinary life. Before Daoists can reach out for the stars, their bodies have to undergo massive transformations and become subtle energy networks. For this, they distinguish different kinds and levels of *qi* in the body.

The most immediately tangible and strongest among them is *jing* 精, often translated "essence." As Manfred Porkert defines it (1974), *jing* is the indeterminate aspect of *qi* or *qi* in transition from one determinate form to another. A classic example is man's semen that carries life from the father to the child; another is the essence that the body takes from food during its assimilation. Neither yin nor yang, *jing* marks *qi* in transit, the raw fuel that drives the pulsating rhythm of the body's cellular reproduction. Governed by the kidneys and the phase water, it is also connected to the primordial *qi* that resides there and to the psychological power of will or determination. It is among the main sources of a person's charisma, sexual attraction, and sense of wholeness.

In its dominant form *jing* is sexual potency, that is, semen in men and menstrual blood in women. Both develop from pure *qi* that sinks down from its center—the Ocean of *Qi* in the abdomen in men and the Cavern of *Qi* in the breast area in women—and becomes tangible in sexual sensations and fluids. Emitting *jing* from the body through untimely ejaculation and excessive menstruation is seen as a major source of *qi*-loss which can cause physical weakness, lead to diseases, and precipitate early death. But even without massive loss of *jing*, vital essence diminishes over a lifetime. Its rise and decline are understood as occurring in an eight-year cycle in males and a seven-year cycle in females, reaching its height as people are in their twenties and thirties and continuously declining until their reproductive functions cease and the body decays in their later years.

The basic concern for all longevity seekers and Daoist practitioners is to regulate and slow down this process of decline, to keep *jing* in the body, and to reverse the downward movement of *qi*. By reverting essence back to *qi* through various physical disciplines and meditation practices, they renew life and enhance vigor, laying the foundation for ultimate energetic refinement.

The *qi* that is at the root of essence and to which it returns in the body is the inner, personal aspect of universal energy. Classified as yang in relation to blood (*xue* 血) as its yin counterpart, this *qi* is made up of both prenatal and postnatal aspects; serves as the foundation of our health and sickness; and determines how we move, eat, sleep, and function in the world. Flowing through the meridians just as blood flows through veins and arteries, it is the source of move-ment in and out of the body, present in continuous circulation.

Also, through breath, food, drink, physical contact, sexuality, and emotions, personal *qi* is in constant exchange with the outside world. As noted earlier, it can be proper, well-aligned, harmonious, right in amount and timing and activity, or wayward, heteropathic, mis-aligned, off-track, and harmful. Practitioners have to make sure their *qi* is proper and flows smoothly. Only the best quality of *qi* should be allowed in the body and only stale, postnatal *qi*, not the valuable pri-mordial part, should be permitted to leave. Adepts develop a high awareness of interaction with the environment as well as great care in the types of food they take and the breathing methods they apply. More and more they learn to focus on the inner patterns and rhythms of *qi*, refining it through continued conscious circulation to subtler and more cosmic levels.

Eventually *qi* is transformed into the finest of internal energies, which flow with the same vibrational frequency as the gods them-selves. The Chinese call this *shen* 神, which means "spirit" as bodily energy but also indicates "gods" and "divine" in religious contexts. Everyone has spirit naturally from birth. Classified as yang, it is the guiding vitality behind the body's senses and the individual's psycho-logical forces, manifesting as individual consciousness and constitut-ing the individual's mental direction. Residing in the heart, it controls the mind and the emotions and through them is an important cause of sickness. Beyond the mind and the emotions, spirit is also the power that connects the person to Heaven and original destiny—an active, organizing configurative force and transformative influence that one cannot perceive directly but only through its manifestations (Kaptchuk 1983, 58).

Adepts strive to transform their *qi* increasingly into spirit, becoming finer and subtler in the basic energetic configuration of their bodies, thereby being more like spirits, gods, and the immortals. Refined in their energetic bodies, they become more aware of the subtler levels of existence, more attuned to the gods, and more potent in their abili-ties. Advanced practitioners not only see and feel the presence of the deities around and within them but also gain various supernatural powers, called aspects of spirit pervasion (*shentong* 神通): they can be in two places at once, move quickly from one place to another, know the past and the future, divine people's thoughts, procure wondrous substances, overcome all hazards of fire and water, and have powers over life and death. Their entire being has shifted from the mundane, *qi*-based world to the realm of the spirit, the divine, the gods. They are firmly on their way of becoming gods themselves (see Despeux and Kohn 2003).

The Present Volume

This book does not concern itself much with these advanced stages. Rather, it focuses on the intermediate level, the stage of the refinement of *qi*, and the various methods by which people can make their energy softer, finer, and subtler to find greater health, higher vitality, extended life expectancy, and an improved awareness of inner energies and outside vibrational patterns. The contributions of the volume are accordingly practical and oriented toward modern application, focusing on the traditional conceptions but dominantly presenting contemporary activities and uses.

This, however, does not mean that this book is a how-to manual. For correct usage of the methods presented, readers should consult a trained professional and take the relevant courses under proper guidance and supervision. Still, they can find inspiration here and learn which Daoist or other kinds of body cultivation might be appropriate for them to enhance life and well-being.

In the first paper, Stockbridge-based acupuncturist and well-known author Lonny Jarrett deals with the medical dimension. He shows how Chinese medicine and acupuncture, when applied with subtlety and energetic awareness, can be powerful instruments in helping people realize their inner authenticity and fulfill their ultimate destiny on the planet. Not only managing symptoms and healing diseases, Chinese medical practice has a spiritual dimension that begins with the manipulation of bodily energies and leads to important spiritual achievements.

Following this, the book focuses on breathing practice. Catherine Despeux, senior researcher at the INALCO Institute in Paris, France, and author of numerous volumes on Chinese religion and longevity, examines the six healing breaths, ways of exhaling with a particular mouth position that will create a certain sound, like *ssss*. Each sound is associated with a particular organ and is said to help with a variety of physical conditions, thus supporting physical health and well-being while increasing the depth of the breath and the awareness of one's breathing patterns. She traces the practice through various forms and sources, finding that it goes back to the beginning of the Common Era and is still very much part of modern Daoism and popular Qigong.

The same holds also true for the practice of *qi*-absorption, studied by Stephen Jackowicz, a trained acupuncturist, Chinese studies Ph. D., and teacher of Chinese medicine in Long Island, New York. As he shows, *qi*-absorption first appears in Han dynasty manuscripts as a method of ingesting *qi*, i.e., eating *qi* instead of food. This method makes the body subtler and independent of outer food but does not transform the digestive system. In contrast, *qi*-absorption involves a connection to the energies of the cosmos and effects a reorganization of the body's energetic system, creating a different physicality in the process. Both methods are used in healing today and represent valid ways of finding well-being and integration.

The same case is also made by Shawn Arthur, assistant professor of Asian Religions at Appalachian State University in Boone, North Carolina. He focuses on the dietary techniques of ancient Daoism and the ways of replacing, reducing, and even stopping all food intake in favor of a higher awareness and the absorption of *qi*. He presents specific recipes of herbal concoctions and alchemical elixirs and outlines their alleged effects. He also recounts testimonies of people who are still actively practicing the ancient dietary regimens today.

Next comes the practice of physical bends and stretches, known as Daoyin and presented by Livia Kohn, professor of Religion and East Asian Studies at Boston University and certified Yoga teacher. Although at first glance very similar to Yoga as it is practiced widely in the West today, Daoyin has its own history, underlying assumptions, and sets of practices that distinguish it thoroughly from Indian methods. Still an active part in contemporary practice, Daoyin has played a role in both the medical and religious communities and been closely connected to breathing techniques, dietary measures, and *qi* absorption.

A more inner focus is the subject of the next contribution by Michael Winn, long-term practitioner of Daoist methods and the leader of Healing Tao, USA. He describes and analyzes the transformation of sexual energies through internal alchemy. First learning to recognize and activate the feeling of *jing* or sexual essence in the body, practitioners reverse its course and mutate it back into *qi*. They then circulate this purified energy through the body and refine it further into pure spirit (*shen*) with the help of water and fire—understood both as alchemical substances and energetic bodily forces. As adepts become more sensitized to their inner energetic structure, they can modify it through careful, gradual practice to a subtler and more spiritual level. Internal alchemy requires an active *qi*-flow, an open body, and a heightened awareness. The various other physical practices are preparatory to it and form a necessary part of its process.

The last two contributions look at Daoist body cultivation in community settings. Bede Bidlack, director of the Still Mountain Tai Chi Center and Ph. D. candidate at Boston College, examines Taiji quan both as a martial art and as a spiritual technique in Daoism. In either role, its movements are practiced in close conjunction with nature and other people. That is to say, one ideally practices outside, in a natural setting, and through the practice develops close awareness of the energetic patterns of nature. Also, one typically practices in groups and learns to maintain constant awareness of what others are doing, a training enhanced in partner practice. Through Taiji quan, therefore, practitioners take their own inner purified *qi* and relate it to the outside world—or, vice versa, they become aware of their *qi* through calm and focused interaction with nature and others, and from there develop a greater urge toward personal refinement.

The last article in the book focuses on Qigong, the modern adaptation of Daoist body cultivation with great popularity in China and increased accessibility in the West. Louis Komjathy, visiting professor at Shandong University, China, looks at its presence in America today, describing its major forms, main representatives, and key characteristics. He points out the role these practices have come to play in our world and how they have been subject to political changes (Chinese communism, American immigration laws) and cultural fads (New Age movement, complementary healthcare). He also notes just to what degree their availability is subject to market factors and how much leading practitioners are ignoring or even distorting historical realities in favor of creating a marketable product.

Daoist body cultivation with its long history and proven efficaciousness can make an important contribution to our stress-ridden, technology-driven world. It can be even more potent if one makes the effort to understand the practices in context, to appreciate the culture from which they came, and to respect their integrity and the demands they may make on becoming a different person: more inward-focused, kinder and gentler, calmer and slower, less consumptive and pleasure-oriented. It may be very rewarding, healthwise and spiritually, to reach out for Daoist attainments, but one should never forget that the traditional goal of the practices is an energetic transfiguration that leads to ultimate transcendence and inner spiritization.

Bibliography

Andersen, Poul. 1994. "The Transformation of the Body in Taoist Ritual." In *Religious Reflections on the Human Body*, edited by Jane Marie Law, 181-202. Bloomington: Indiana University Press.

Bumbacher, Stephan Peter. 2001. "Zu den Körpergottheiten im chinesischen Taoismus." In *Noch eine Chance für die Religionsphänomenologie?*, edited by D. Peoli-Olgiati, A. Michaels, and F. Stolz, 151-72. Frankfurt: Peter Lang.

Despeux, Catherine. 2005. "Visual Representations of the Body in Chinese Medical and Daoist Texts from the Song to the Qing." *Asian Medicine—Tradition and Modernity* 1: 10-52

_____, and Livia Kohn. 2003. *Women in Daoism*. Cambridge, Mass.: Three Pines Press.

Homann, Rolf. 1971. *Die wichtigsten Körpergottheiten im Huang-t'ing-ching*. Göppingen: Alfred Kümmerle.

Ishida, Hidemi. 1989. "Body and Mind: The Chinese Perspective." In *Taoist Meditation and Longevity Techniques*, edited by Livia Kohn, 41-70. Ann Arbor: University of Michigan, Center for Chinese Studies Publications.

Kaptchuk, Ted J. 1983. *The Web that Has No Weaver: Understanding Chinese Medicine*. New York: Congdon & Weed.

Kohn, Livia. 1991. "Taoist Visions of the Body." *Journal of Chinese Philosophy* 18: 227-52.

_____. 1995. *Laughing at the Tao: Debates among Buddhists and Taoists in Medieval China*. Princeton: Princeton University Press.

_____. 2005. *Health and Long Life: The Chinese Way*. Cambridge, Mass.: Three Pines Press.

Komjathy, Louis. 2002. *Title Index to Daoist Collections*. Cambridge, Mass.: Three Pines Press.

Kroll, Paul W. 1996. "Body Gods and Inner Vision: *The Scripture of the Yellow Court*. In *Religions of China in Practice*, edited by Donald S. Lopez Jr., 149-55. Princeton: Princeton University Press.

Lincoln, Bruce. 1975. "The Indo-European Myth of Creation." *History of Religions* 15: 121-45.

Major, John S. 1978. "Myth, Cosmology, and the Origins of Chinese Science." *Journal of Chinese Philosophy* 5: 1-20.

Porkert, Manfred. 1974. *The Traditional Foundations of Chinese Medicine*. Cambridge, Mass.: MIT Press.

Robinet, Isabelle. 1993. *Taoist Meditation*. Translated by Norman Girardot and Julian Pas. Albany: State University of New York Press.

Saso, Michael. 1997. "The Taoist Body and Cosmic Prayer." In *Religion and the Body*, edited by Sarah Coakley, 231-47. Cambridge: Cambridge University Press.

Schipper, Kristofer M. 1978. "The Taoist Body." *History of Religions* 17: 355-87.

_____. 1994. *The Taoist Body*. Translated by Karen C. Duval. Berkeley: University of California Press.

_____, and Franciscus Verellen, eds. 2004. *The Taoist Canon: A Historical Companion to the Daozang*. 3 vols. Chicago: University of Chicago Press.

Ware, James R. 1966. *Alchemy, Medicine and Religion in the China of A.D. 320*. Cambridge, Mass.: MIT Press.

Chapter One

Acupuncture and Spiritual Realization

LONNY JARRETT

> The upper [class of] medicines govern the nourishment of
> destiny and correspond to Heaven. . . . If one wishes to pro-
> long the years of life without aging, one should [use these].
>
> The middle [class of] medicines govern the nourishment of
> one's nature and correspond to man. . . . If one wishes to
> prevent illness and to supplement depletions and emacia-
> tions, one should [use these].
>
> The lower [class of] medicines . . . govern the treatment of
> illness and correspond to earth. If one wishes to remove cold,
> heat and [other] evil influences [from the body], to break ac-
> cumulations, and to cure illnesses, one should base [one's ef-
> forts] on [drugs listed in] the lower [class of this] manual.
> (*Shenong bencao jing*)

This passage is from the *Shenong bencao jing* 神農本草經 (The Divine
Farmer's Materia Medica), China's oldest herbal text and a work that
goes back to Han origins. Lost early, it was reconstituted by the Daoist master Tao Hongjing 陶弘景 (456-536) from fragments and citations and contains over 700 drugs in the three classes described. It is
very clear in this passage that the highest aspect of healing involves
helping the patient fulfill his or her destiny in order to live out the
years allotted by Heaven.

Below that level of healing is the nourishment of people's inherent
nature or constitution (*xing* 性). The lowest class of medicine treats
only physical illness. As early as the fourth century C.E., the alchemist Ge Hong 葛洪 in his *Baopuzi* 抱朴子 (Book of the Master Who
Embraces Simplicity, DZ 1185) laments that these words come from

19

the highest sages, yet the people of his age have lost their belief in the efficacy of the highest forms of medicine (Ware 1966, 177).

The human body is the primary vehicle for the evolution of conscious-ness and spirit. From the perspective of deep time, it has taken nearly fourteen billion years for Dao to cultivate matter to the degree of complexity that is evident in human form to support the emergence of self-reflective consciousness. Yet, Dao awakens to its own nature only through the awakening of the human mind. The highest purpose of medicine in this context is to remove all impediments that inhibit this. Cultivation exercises can support the process of awakening, but it is always consciousness, intention, and purity of motive that are primary in the realization of our shared human destiny (*ming* 命) in attaining enlightenment (*ming* 明) or self-realization. The process of physical healing or strengthening the body through the practice of medicine must always be considered to be of secondary importance to these highest goals which do not necessarily take time except for our own resistance and disinterest in attaining them.

In my writings I have delineated an inner tradition of Chinese medi-cine, whose primary therapeutic focus is to help patients fulfill their personal destiny (see Jarrett 1999; 2003). The term "inner tradition" refers to the practice of Chinese medicine in a way that places pri-mary emphasis on the use of medicine as a tool to aid spiritual evolu-tion. Most notably, a patient's progress in treatment is assessed by indicators of conscious awareness and a balanced relationship to the presence of thought and feeling rather than, as is done in more exter-nal traditions of practice, assessing response to treatment with pri-mary emphasis on the relative presence or absence of pain or other physical symptoms. Of course, inherent in the inner tradition is the expectation that physical symptoms will improve as the constitu-tional or karmic basis of illness is resolved at a deep level.

The inner tradition is most explicitly concerned with the psycho-spiritual basis of illness and views physical symptoms and signs as relatively superficial manifestations which are compensations for un-derlying constitutional issues. This view is expressed in the *Shennong bencao jing,* which matches the treatment of physical illness to the lowest class of medicine. This is also a key understanding in Daoism, as is made clear in a statement by Liu Cao 劉操, traditionally the teacher of Zhang Boduan 張伯端 (983-1082) and Wang Chongyang 王重陽 (1113-1171), founders of the Southern and Northern schools of Complete Perfection (Quanzhen 全真) Daoism:

> If the basic energy is not stabilized, the spirit is insecure.
> Let insects eat away at the root of a tree, and the leaves dry
> up. Stop talking about mucus, saliva, semen, and blood—
> when you get to the basis and find out the original source,
> they are all the same. When has this thing ever had a fixed
> location? It changes according to the time, according to mind
> and ideas. (Cleary 1989, xxvi)

Another hallmark of the inner tradition is that it explicitly serves as
an extension of the practitioner's own spiritual quest and path. The
diagnostics inherent in the inner tradition require the practitioner to
listen with all senses and with increasingly deeper sensitivity to the
cues that spontaneously emerge from the patient. This method of
honing the senses may, in time, clear away the accretions of experience and interpretation that color the practitioner's own perception of
reality. Thus, through discipline and attentive practice, the heart and
mind of the practitioner may be reunited. One's efficacy as a healer
lies in large part in having become one's art. And, of course, a practitioner cannot engender a virtue in a patient to any greater degree
than he or she has authentically embraced it.

In the following, I will examine Chinese medicine and its potential for
aiding the spiritual development for both patient and practitioner.
The discussion will focus on five phases constitutional medicine as a
basis for the rediscovery of authentic spontaneity in Dao. But first we
turn our attention to the nature of the path itself.

The Loss and Return of Spontaneity

The Daoist view of our spiritual progression through life can be simply described as a human being's loss of and return to spontaneity
(*ziran* 自然), the original so-being in the Dao (Jarrett 1999, 87-102).
At the moment of conception, Heaven is thought to invest the light of
destiny in each human being as his or her complement of the Three
Treasures: *jing* 精 (essence), *qi* 氣 (energy), and *shen* 神 (spirit). These
three influences guide the development of the fetus, infant, and young
child in a way that ensures the expression of Heaven's will in the
world. At these early stages of development, life is conceived as being
a pure expression of Dao reflecting the fundamental integrity of the
primordial influences. This fundamental state of unity with Dao, then,
is the basis of the ultimate spontaneity and authenticity of the person,
the way he or she can be most authentic (*zhen* 真) in this life.

The *Daode jing* 道德經 (Book of the Dao and Its Virtue) tells us in its first sentence that the Dao that can be named is not the eternal Dao. The emergence of all creation occurs at the moment Dao initiates its movement toward self-consciousness. In the ontogeny of the human being, this is the moment of birth—not the child's physical birth, but the birth of self-awareness. The seeds of self-awareness are sown when the infant receives a name in the third month of life, i.e., one year after conception. The act of receiving a personal name differentiates the infant from all the other people and things—much as in Daoist cosmology the two are differentiated from the one to become the ten thousand things.

Named, the infant grows into a child, creating a false sense of personhood based on individuation and separation from the flowing unity inherent in its primordial being. The momentum supporting this sense of separation develops as we habitually interpret our life experience and our thoughts and feelings in a personal context, which we create in denial of our fundamental oneness with Dao as the source of all manifestations. For, in truth, humans are merely vehicles through which the Dao learns about itself and the experience of life is, at its heart, not personal. As feelings of separation grow, inherent nature or virtue (*de* 德) is lost and spontaneous authenticity dwindles.

Life is now seen through a screen that filters out all information and experience in conflict either with our created self-image or with our perspective on the very nature of life itself. This is clearly expressed by Liu Yiming 劉一明, an important nineteenth-century interpreter of Daoist and Buddhist esoteric writing whose work illuminates the spiritual and psychological significance of Chinese physiology and the inner traditions of Chinese medicine. He says,

> Man gradually grows from childhood . . . yin and yang divide, each dwelling on one side, in the center of truth there is artificiality. Here knowledge and experience gradually develop, and good and bad are discriminated.[1]

It is a matter of destiny that oneness with Dao is lost as the child becomes a fundamentally divided human being. This fundamental division of yin and yang represents a crack in the very foundation and

---

[1] See Liu's commentary on Zhang Boduan' alchemical text, *Jindan sibai zi* 金丹四百字 (Four Hundred Characters Explaining the Golden Elixir), and his own work *Duanpo yanyi* 斷破言疑 (Symbolic Language: Breaking Open Doubt). For an English translation, see Cleary 1986.

root of life. From a spiritual perspective, it is the engine that drives susceptibility to all the syndrome patterns in Chinese medicine and the separation of the five phases. In alchemical terms, yin denotes the false, created, self or ego whereas yang denotes the authentic spontaneity that arises out of the primordial influences of *jing*, *qi*, and *shen*. A general principle of medicine is to remove stagnation before tonifying. And what greater stagnation could there be in life than having forgotten one's inherent nature as an expression of Dao?

The path to illness is predicated upon building a self through one choice and one action at a time, a self that is experienced as being separate, not only from all other manifest things but from Dao as the unborn source of life itself.[2] The path of healing is one of reintegration. It is in our own recognition that we have moved away from inherent nature and our single pointed intention to return back to a state of flowing oneness that transforms the latent potential or essence and inherent nature of the infant into the illuminated virtue of the sage.[3]

The Five Phases

Chinese medicine includes twelve diagnostic methods that elaborate the quality of an individual's functional separation from Dao. Among them, the number one corresponds to the recognition of the underlying oneness that is a continual expression of Dao uncolored by an independent sense of self. The number two allows us to assess the separation of yin and yang, the not-real from the real, as the engine that drives all functional disharmony. At this foundational level the purpose of medicine is to remove what is false and strengthen the influence of what is real.

The number eight, a higher order expression of two and the foundation of the eight-principle system of Chinese diagnostics, allows us to assess how the false has become physiologically and structurally em-

---

[2] The ultimate black and white nature of our choices as empowering either yin/ mundaneness or yang/life is illustrated in the transition from hexagram 23 to 24 of the *Yijing* 易經 (Book of Changes). For a discussion, see Jarrett 1999, 103-17.

[3] The name Laozi 老子 literally means old infant. The *Daode jing* instructs us on the preservation of original nature and its transformation into virtue denoted by the same character, *de*. For a further discussion of *de*, see Jarrett 1999, 45 and 358-59.

bodied as functional and physical pathology.[4] All stagnations dis-
cussed in Chinese medicine such as stagnant blood, *qi*, wind, cold,
heat, and dampness, or the presence of dryness can be considered to
be the physiological correlates of separation and delusion.

The number five, as present in the five phases model, allows us to
elaborate the quality of an individual's destiny and path of healing as
an expression of Heaven and yang. Hence we may discern the degree
to which the absolute nature of spirit is expressed in consciousness as
reflected in words and deeds. We may also appreciate the degree to
which perception and behavior are distorted and conditioned by
weather, thoughts, and feelings, all of which are differentiated according to the five phases model. As Liu Yiming describes the workings of the five phases:

> When yin and yang divide, the five phases become disor-
> dered. The five phases—metal, wood, water, fire, and
> earth—represent the five *qi*. The five phases of pre-Heaven
> [primordiality] create each other following the productive
> cycle. These five phases fuse to form a unified *qi*. From them
> issue forth the five virtues of benevolence, righteousness,
> propriety, wisdom, and integrity. [The five phases] of post-
> Heaven [mundaneness] overcome one another following the
> controlling cycle. This manifests as the five rebels of joy, an-
> ger, grief, happiness, and desire.
>
> When the five phases are united, the five virtues are pre-
> sent and yin and yang form a chaotic unity. Once the five
> phases divide, the distinguishing spirit gradually arises,
> and the encrustation of the senses gradually takes place;
> truth flees and the false becomes established. Now, even the
> state of the child is lost. (*Jindan sibai zijie*; Cleary 1986)

Although several of the relations found in five phases theory (such as
the five planets and five directions) appear in records of the Shang
dynasty (ca. 1600-1028 B.C.E.), the five phases system was not fully
elaborated until about 350 B.C.E., when it was formulated by the cos-
mologist Zou Yan 鄒衍 (Kaptchuk 1983, 345). The language used by
the early Chinese to describe their world is one of poetic images rich
in associative value. Water names the phase associated with winter
because of its tendency to freeze and become focused in that season.
Wood names the phase associated with spring because it grows rap-

---

[4] See Jarrett 2003, ch. 37 for a detailed comparison of the five-phases
and eight-principle systems. Note that in Chinese numerology even numbers
are yin in nature and odd numbers are yang.

idly at that time of year. Fire names the phase associated with summer because of the increased heat during those months when the sun reaches its zenith. Earth names the phase associated with late summer, as the fields are abundant then with the fruit of earth's bounty. Metal names the phase associated with fall as the farmer's knife reaps the harvest of that season.

In their natural rhythm, the five phases produce each other continuously in a harmonious cycle. Thus, water comes about through rainfall. It makes things grow, so that there is lush vegetation and wood arises. Wood dries and becomes fuel for fire, which burns and creates ashes. Ashes become earth, and earth over long periods of consolidation grows metals in its depths. Metals in the depths of mountains, moreover, attract clouds and stimulate rainfall, thus closing the productive cycle.

At the same time, however, the five phases also work in mutual control, keeping things in their proper order. Thus, water can extinguish fire, fire can melt metal, metal can cut wood, wood can contain earth, earth can dam water, and water can again extinguish fire. Here the inherently dynamic nature of the five phases is not used to increase productivity, but to set boundaries and limit potential excesses in what is know as the controlling cycle.

These laws governing nature's dynamic process of change were codified over thousands of years. The system of the five transformations provides a qualitative standard of reference to which we may refer all observations regarding the functional dynamics of all phenomena.[5] Daoists viewed humans as microcosms of the universe, and the five phases system allows for the assessment of each individual's relationship to his or her own inner nature as well as to the surrounding world. Five phases theory describes the character and relationships of the identifiable functions comprising human nature. The associations of the five phases system allow us to qualitatively assess an individual's relative degree of functional balance through the interpretation of signs that emanate continually with every form of personal expression.

In the five phases system, each individual is believed to have a constitutional tendency to emulate the quality of expression of one season

---

[5] See Jarrett 1999, 435-53 for a detailed comparison of the cognitive styles inherent in Chinese medicine and Western medicine.

of the year more than others.[6] The natural qualities of this season are thought to define an individual's inherited weaknesses and strengths. Some associations of each phase are listed below.

The Basic Associations of the Five Phases

phase	color	sound	odor	emotion	weather	virtue
water	blue	groan	putrid	fear	cold	wisdom
wood	green	shout	rancid	anger	wind	benevolence
fire	red	laugh	scorched	joy	heat	propriety
earth	yellow	sing	fragrant	worry	dampness	integrity
metal	white	weep	rotten	grief	dryness	righteous-ness

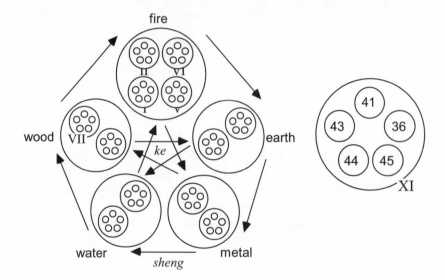

Fig. 1: The exchange patterns of the five phases.

In its most basic form, the tradition elaborates the five broad movements of Dao into twelve main organs and meridians, the relative balance of which constitute the dynamic web of the productive and controlling cycles (see Fig. 1).

---

[6] The concept of the five-phases constitutional types is presented in chapter 64 of the *Huangdi neijing lingshu* 黃帝內經靈樞 (The Yellow Emperor's Inner Classic, Numinous Pivot). For a translation, see Ki 1985; Wu 1993.

The first part of Figure 1 shows the five phases in their productive and controlling cycles. Each organ is depicted in the order of *qi*-flow according to the Chinese clock beginning with the heart, i.e., "fire" at the top of the diagram. The phases create each other following the productive (*sheng*) cycle and limit each other according to the controlling (*ke*) cycle. They each match certain of the twelve main organs corresponding to the yin and yang aspects of the phases.[7] Each aspect, therefore, retains its own discrete function yet has within it the implicit representation of the whole cycle.

This representation is present most actively at the acupuncture points of each meridian that are associated with the various phases. The second part of Figure 1 provides an example. It shows the five phases points on the stomach meridian, which begins below the pupils, passes across the head, moves down through the torso, stomach, and groin, continues along the outside of the legs, and ends at the second toe. On this meridian, which has a total of forty-five points, St-41 is the fire point and relates to the heart, St-36 is the earth point that relates to the spleen, and so forth.

The productive cycle names the order in which the phases produce or give birth to each other. The water phase, therefore, may be said to give birth to the wood phase along this cycle. This sequence is the natural order that the seasons create during the year. The controlling cycle gives the order in which the phases limit or control each other. Thus water may be said to control fire across the controlling cycle. An example of this relationship between water and fire is that the potential present in any seed (water) always limits the maximum height (fire) a tree may attain given the best possible environment.

In a state of functional balance, the phases produce and limit each other effortlessly. When *qi* stops flowing in its natural progression around the productive cycle and becomes fixed in its expression, the phases begin to block each other through the controlling cycle, resulting in chaos and eventually illness. In other words, *qi* that travels along the controlling cycle and is termed aggressive energy may form the basis of serious pathology, such as cancer, heart disease, and mental illness (Jarrett 2003, 16-36). Liu Yiming refers to this pre-

---

[7] The twelve main organs and meridians and their phase associations (yin/yang) are: fire—heart, small intestine, heart protector, triple heater; earth—spleen, stomach; metal—lungs, large intestine; water—kidneys, bladder; and wood—liver, gallbladder. They form the backbone of Chinese medicine. In the *Huangdi neijing* (ch. 8), they are moreover personified as officials, each in charge of specific functions. See Larre and Rochat de la Valle 1986.

dicament and describes how the five phases separate as a conse-
quence of the fundamental division of yin and yang at the root.

In addition to phase type, each person's constitution is assessed according to the dictates of a particular organ system, each of which has
many discrete aspects of function. These are accessible through the
acupuncture points on the organ's related meridian, yet also contain
the implicit presence of the other phases and functions (Jarrett 1999,
130-35).

Constitutional Types

Each individual sees life through a filter determined by the domi-
nance of one of the five phases. This filtration is in itself impersonal.
That is to say, from the black and white perspective of yin and yang
the separate sense of ego functions exactly the same in everyone. On
the other hand, the qualitative nature of this screen can be differentiated according to a patient's inborn nature or five phases constitutional type.

According to this model, each person embodies the quality of expression that is present during one season more than the others. This
phase is the patient's constitutional type and provides a framework
for organizing observations of how the patient has come to embody
his or her interpretation of life in every aspect of being. Constitutional type may be thought of as the tint on the window through
which people observe life, the coloring and filter of their interpretation of everything they see and experience. Recognizing a patient's
basic constitutional type allows the practitioner to see into his or her
depths, through the accretions of acquired experience, and back toward the source. It allows us to determine the specific way that each
individual embodies the meaning he or she attributes to life and thus
helps us understand how the patient has lost touch with inner authenticity. It also provides a framework for determining the steps
that need to be taken to restore inherent nature.

At its core, each of the five phases has a quality of destiny that en-
compasses the process of life transformation for individuals manifesting the corresponding constitutional type. This process involves
transforming our habituated relationship to the presence of emotions
and thoughts into one of objectivity on our internal experience. As we
become free in the face of our experience, spontaneity is restored, and

the virtue corresponding to our constitutional type is engendered. This complex process can be graphically depicted by showing the virtue of each phase in the center and the effects of excess and deficient emotional reaction to the left and right.

In the chart below, the five phases appear on the same vertical line as the personal attributes or virtues that emerge when the destiny of a specific constitutional type is being fulfilled. As a given virtue erodes, on the other hand, a habitually occurring behavior arises depending on the presence of an excessive or diminished emotion, listed on the horizontal plane.

Water

WISDOM

excessive fear	deficient caution
conservativeness	recklessness
orthodoxy	fantasy
stinginess	profligacy
dormancy	scatteredness

Fire

PROPRIETY

excessive joy	deficient enthusiasm
control	chaos
tyranny	sycophantism
guardedness	vulnerability
delusion	dullness

Wood

BENEVOLENCE

excessive anger	deficient drive
belligerence	timidity
resentment	indecision
arrogance	humility
determination	resignation

Metal

RIGHTEOUSNESS

excessive longing	deficient courage
gain	loss
fullness	emptiness
materialism	asceticism
vanity	self-depreciation

Earth

INTEGRITY/HONESTY

excessive worry	deficient sympathy
self-indulgence	ingratiation
selfishness	martyrdom
self-sufficiency	neediness
obsession	boredom

For example, someone who is constitutionally a water-type, given any major stress in life, will interpret what is happening according to the associations of water and react emotionally with fear or caution. As the habitual presence or lack of this dominant attitude increases, there is a corresponding erosion of the inherent water-virtue of wisdom. The person becomes more limited in his or her choices and works herself into a particular corner of being.

On the other hand, it is her life destiny to consciously strive toward manifesting wisdom as the virtue corresponding to her constitutional type and to overcome her innate pattern of reaction with fear and/or caution. The one to attain full realization is the Daoist sage, often metaphorically depicted with a large skull to show that he has overcome fear and transformed essence into marrow, brain, bone, and wisdom. Note also that when any one virtue is manifest, they are all manifest. For example, having integrity, the virtue ascribed to earth, implies the presence of wisdom, benevolence, propriety, and righteousness, the virtues of the other phases.

In monitoring a patient's progress in treatment, the practitioner must focus on transforming the primary disordered emotion and resulting habitual behavior back into their corresponding virtue. For example, if the patient responds habitually to avoid the emotion longing or sadness and lacks courage in life, then various behaviors leading to gain and loss may be displayed. If the patient can remain in the presence of the emotion and not let it dictate his or her actions, then the corresponding virtue of righteousness is empowered. To remain in the presence of an emotion, no matter how powerful, and make the right choices is a profound manifestation of liberation. The skilled practitioner is able to test the patient's emotions both during the intake and throughout the course of treatment in order to determine if they are functioning more appropriately over time. A positive shift in the patient's emotive state toward the emergence of a given virtue always indicates that healing is occurring on the deepest level as the primordial *qi* reasserts its influence in the patient's life.

Understanding the associations of the five phases model thus offers a perspective to see through relative conditioning, to understand patterns of habituated behavior, and to see back toward the source of being. Many practitioners think that the primary purpose of the five phases model is to help harmonize patients with the seasonal flow of *qi*. For them, the goal of treatment is to free a person to move along with the seasons of life so that he or she is no longer stuck in the expression of any one phase.

However, due in large part to the fact that Chinese medicine was assimilated into the West in the 1970s, at a time when humanist psychology was ascendant in popularity, they commonly miss the more spiritual point of the model. This point is that, from the absolute perspective of spiritual attainment, the ultimate goal of the practice is not merely to reside in harmony with the flow of *qi* in the productive cycle but rather to transcend it in favor of oneness with Dao. In other words, residing in harmony with the phases is too often synonymous with the idea of going into and processing one's thoughts and feelings. The true goal of medicine and Daoist body cultivation, on the other hand, is to empower freedom from thoughts and feelings and not identification with them.

The Sanskrit term *samsāra* denotes the state of continuous reincarnation due to being lost in illusion and ignorance. The Chinese translation of *samsāra* consists of the words "life" (*sheng* 生) and "death" (*si* 死). Thus, someone caught in a state of *samsāra* is trapped in an endless cycle of life and death or death and rebirth. The productive or "life" (*sheng*) cycle of the five phases, denoting the endless transformation of one into another, in one sense depicts this predicament. To the degree that the phases are conditioned by ego, the productive cycle is a habituated circle of identification with conditioned thought/feeling on the inside and climate/weather on the outside— representing the internal and external causes of disease.

Each position of the phase points on the productive cycle represents the relative position of the constitutional type. In its greatest detail, a patient's constitution may be said to be fire within wood, water within earth, or any of the other possibilities (Jarrett 2003, ch. 12). Each type, moreover, represents the personal perspective of the individual on his or her life experience as assimilated through the window of his constitution.

From the perspective of the center of the circle, the Taiji 太極 or Great Ultimate, on the other hand, each constitutional type generates illness because it represents a movement away from oneness with Dao. This movement has occurred through a process of personalizing life experience to build a separate sense of self, a process that denies our fundamental nature of unity with each other and all things to which Dao gives birth. Although each relative position has its own unique physiological attributes that can be differentiated and addressed through the practice of Chinese medicine, the step back to the absolute center of the circle is the same for each of us. This step involves the one-pointed focus on discovering the true nature of who we are and why we are here. It is a step that ultimately takes no time at all as it only ever involves acknowledging what is already true right now. It means the discovery of a self-nature that is continually developmental and not ultimately conditioned or limited by our emergence into being on planet Earth with its repetitive seasonal movements.

The Application of Medicine

Each acupuncture point is unique in its ability to touch some aspect of being that has been lost to the individual. By touching this aspect, the memory of inherent, spontaneous nature encoded within the point's function may be restored to the patient. Acupuncture points work by harmonizing continuums of unbalanced and extreme expressions back into the virtues from which they derive. They revitalize patients by drawing on a source of pure *qi*, a source rooted in Dao as the unborn ground of our being, a source that is untouched by the vicissitudes of life. The following case history illustrates this point.

Lynda was a 31-year-old woman who came to receive help with migraine headaches. These always presented on the outside margin of her right orbit in the location of the first point of the gallbladder meridian, located near the eyes and called Pupil Bone (Tongziliao 瞳子髎, Gb-1). She sighed constantly and was hopeless regarding the completion of her doctoral thesis and the stress it was putting on her relationship with her fiancé. Her liver pulse was tense and she reported feeling tension in the diaphragm right near the acupuncture point Gate of Hope (Qimen 期門, Lv-14).

According to my analysis, Lynda was a wood constitutional type as evidenced by her greenish color, the sound of her sighing, her slightly rancid odor, and her suppressed anger. Her headaches at the beginning of the gallbladder meridian and the pressure felt at Gate of Hope on the liver meridian both suggested *qi*-stagnation as the result of a dysfunctional wood-phase. This finding was supported by her tense liver pulse and her constant sighing which can be interpreted as the venting of frustration and a sign of liver-*qi* stagnation. Her state of hopelessness can be interpreted as the liver inhibiting the flow of *qi* across the diaphragm area so that it fails to support the function of the heart and lungs whose virtues include compassion and inspiration respectively.

The treatment I provided began with activating the liver meridian by needling Insect Drain (Ligou 蠡溝, Lv-5), a connecting point that unites the function of the liver with that of the gallbladder. The name "Insect Drain" refers to this point's ability to help the liver detoxify the blood whose function it is to empower us to feel comfortable inside ourselves. The point also helps us hold a bigger perspective in the face of annoying details. To supplement this, I then needled Gate of Hope, which helps to relieve *qi*-stagnation in the diaphragm area and to empower the positive force of hopefulness.

On the gallbladder meridian, I worked with its source point Wilderness Mount (Qiuxu 邱墟, Gb-40). A source point is a point near the wrist or ankle where the source-*qi* of the meridian flows most clearly and where it is retained and strengthened most easily. The source point on the gallbladder meridian empowers the virtue of perspective. In addition, I used Pupil Bone, located on the outer corner of the eye right in the area of Lynda's headaches. This enhances clarity of vision and, in this case, reinforced the intention of treating Wilderness Mount.

In addition, I also treated Dove Tail (*Jiuwei* 鳩尾, CV-15) on the Conception Vessel, the channel that runs straight up the center of the torso from the pubic area to the nostrils. Located in the lower chest area, this is the wood-phase (i.e., liver-connected) point of the heart protector meridian. It renews the heart by providing access to a clear source of *qi*. It also helps to open up the diaphragm area in conjunction with Gate of Hope. The last point I inserted a needle in was Inner Frontier (Neiguan 內關, HP-6) on the heart protector meridian, a yang energy line that supports the heart and runs up from the hands along the outside of the arm. In conjunction with Gate of Hope and Dove Tail, it works to relieve tension in the diaphragm and allows *qi* to enter the domain of the heart, the "inner frontier."

The treatment consisted in retaining all needles for twenty minutes during which Lynda was left to relax on the treatment table alone. Upon returning I asked her what her experience was and she stated: "I am so much more relaxed. I can see how I have been taking my frustration out on my fiancé. It is as though a veil has been lifted from my eyes, like I can finally see the forest for the trees." Within several treatments Lynda's headaches were much improved and her sighing and the tension in her diaphragm region disappeared completely. She also stopped expressing victimization regarding her thesis and the project came to a conclusion with much greater ease.

It is an interesting phenomenon that the function of the acupuncture points is literally encoded within them. I find this confirmed whenever a patient speaks directly to the functions of the points and the intention of the treatment without any prior knowledge regarding the nature of the selected points.

Often, when I return to the treatment room, the patient awakes from the treatment startled without recognizing where he is, whether or not the needles are still in, or how long he has been lying there. When this occurs, acupuncture has given the patient an experience of spontaneity beyond mind, time, and space—mind being an evolutionary adaptation that allows human beings to negotiate their way in the realm of time and space and as such different from pure consciousness. Mind in fact is the facility that becomes conditioned by life experience to ultimately delude consciousness itself.

The state experienced by the patient beyond space-time and mind, then, is full of the latent potential of Dao to create something from nothing. In this state the patient may glimpse original spontaneity in a state of authenticity that is never touched by ordinary life experience and always exists beyond the conditioned mind. The realization may come that, in relation to life's perceived traumas, nothing actually ever happened. Hence we may cease to be the victims of the mind's conclusions and of thoughts and feelings as we take a step back to the center of the circle, a step toward transcendence and the ultimate freedom of Dao.

The habituated momentum that supports the created self is strong and easily reasserts itself. In Western consumer society, patients often seek relief from suffering or experiences of higher states with no desire to change their lives, the very lives that led to illness in the first place. It is important that the practitioner has the skill, experience, and interest to reinforce the positive momentum initiated by the treatment. If we are to make the greatest possible difference, it will be necessary for the patient to allow the states that he or she experiences from treatment to become the basis of new life stages. Healing thus means moving to a higher stage of development that is more or less successful depending on both the patient's own will and the clarity of the practitioner's intention. And the practitioner can only motivate the patient to strive toward higher and more integrated states to the degree that this striving is present at the core of the practitioner's own life.

Conclusion

Roughly fourteen billion years ago something came forth from nothing. This event most certainly represents a giant "Yes!" on the part of that unborn nameless ground of being that Laozi termed "eternal Dao." This ultimate positivity and interest in becoming ever more and more is the nature of that central axis of life itself. The ceaseless striving of the first cause has evolved matter to arrive at the most complex and integrated form that we know of in this universe, the human body and nervous system. Being part of matter, we humans created the Hubble telescope allowing us to peer into infinity and back toward the moment of our own genesis. Looking through that telescope at the yin-yang spiral galaxies, 100 billion at last count, we humans are literally the universe waking up to, and discovering, its own developmental nature. "Oh my!" consciousness says, "Look who I am, look what I've done!" For the founders of Chinese medicine, being one with nature meant living in harmony with the earth's seasonal transitions. I wonder, in the context of our greatly expanded view of nature today, what it might mean to realize our oneness with those hundred billion galaxies and the evolutionary impulse that puts them and us here now.

Through the awakening human being, Dao comes home to itself as Heaven and Earth, and the manifest and latent realms realize their unity at the level of consciousness. It is the highest purpose of medicine to liberate *qi* to flow in this ever upward evolutionary spiral. And humans are the only species that can self-direct their evolution through the inner alchemy that applies the conscious exertion of will and the application of interest. While physical cultivation can strengthen and harmonize the vessel, consciousness awakening to itself is the only true medicine.[8]

Bibiliography

Cleary, Thomas. 1986. *The Inner Teachings of Taoism*. Boston: Shambhala.

_____. 1989. *The Book of Balance and Harmony: Chung He Chi*. San Francisco: North Point Press.

Jarrett, Lonny S. 1999. *Nourishing Destiny: The Inner Tradition of Chinese Medicine*. Stockbridge, Mass.: Spirit Path Press.

_____. 2003. *The Clinical Practice of Chinese Medicine*. Stockbridge, Mass.: Spirit Path Press.

Kaptchuk, Ted J. 1983. *The Web that Has No Weaver: Understanding Chinese Medicine*. New York: Congdon & Weed.

Ki, Sunu. 1985. *The Canon of Acupuncture: Huangti Nei Ching Ling Shu*. Los Angeles: Yuin University Press.

Larre, Claude, J. Schatz, E. Rochat, and S. Stang. 1986. *Survey of Traditional Chinese Medicine*. Paris: Institut Ricci.

Ware, James R. 1966. *Alchemy, Medicine and Religion in the China of AD 320*. Cambridge, Mass.: MIT Press.

Wu, Jing-Nuan. 1993. *Ling Shu or The Spiritual Pivot*. Washington, D.C.: The Taoist Center.

---

[8] I highly recommend reading the journal *What Is Enlightenment?* for a post-postmodern survey of evolutionary enlightenment. See www.wie.org.

Chapter Two

The Six Healing Breaths

CATHERINE DESPEUX[1]

Ever since antiquity, breathing exercises have held a prominent place among the arts of nourishing life and have played an important role in Daoist body cultivation. Many texts describe a particular breathing technique know as the "method of the six breaths" (*liuqi fa* 六氣法) or the "formula of the six characters" (*liuzi jue* 六字訣). The technique has numerous variations and in some forms is still part of contemporary Qigong practice as well as of various Daoist schools, including the methods of inner alchemy as taught by Mantak Chia in the Healing Tao (see Kim 1979; Chia and Chia 1993, 104-05).

What, then, are the six healing breaths? Part of the larger practice of healing exercises (*daoyin* 導引), the absorption of *qi* (*fuqi* 服氣), and the meditative guiding of *qi* (*xingqi* 行氣), they are six ways of exhaling the breath in a particular manner, each described by a Chinese character. In Chinese history, many different breathing methods were developed: in and out through either nose or mouth, in through one and out through the other. Whichever way it was used, however, breathing has always been a central feature of cultivation practice.[2]

---

[1] This contribution is an expanded translation of Despeux 1995. It was translated and supplemented by Livia Kohn.

[2] Ute Engelhardt distinguishes four modes of breathing in Qigong: natural or harmonious (abdominal) breathing, techniques emphasizing exhalation, those emphasizing inhalation, and methods that encourage holding the breath. The first two are most common in Qigong practice today, with natural breathing being the more elementary method and exhalation emphasis—including the six healing breaths—belonging to more advanced levels (1996, 20-22).

In this context it may well have served a certain exorcistic function, not unlike the ancient magic of "whistling" which was used before the Han dynasty to evoke the spirits of the wind, rain, clouds, and thunder, but also demons and goblins. Later whistling became a vocal art, practiced either as a long expiration through narrowed and rounded lips, a vocalization with lips kept open, or a whistling on two fingers (see Sawada 1974).

The earliest mention of breathing practice, including also some of the characters used for the six healing breaths, appears in the *Zhuangzi* 莊子 (Book of Zhuangzi) of the fourth century B.C.E. The text says:

> To huff and puff, exhale and inhale, blow out the old and draw in the new, do the "bear-hang" and the "bird-stretch," interested only in long life—such are the tastes of the practitioners of "guide-and-pull" [*daoyin*] exercises, the nurturers of the body, Grandfather Peng's ripe-old-agers. (ch. 15; Graham 1986, 265)

Rather denigrating in tone, the passage serves to extol the superior methods of mind cultivation and ecstatic travels which allow practitioners to reach the higher realms of heaven. Still, it is interesting in that it uses the various classical terms for breathing practice. "Huff and puff" translates *chuixu* 吹呴, both words used among the six healing breaths where they describe a hot and a cold breath, done with open and closed mouth, respectively. "Exhale and inhale" is *huxi* 呼吸, a binome that begins with exhalation because that is considered the yang part of the process, the movement of the breath being up and outward. The word *hu*, moreover, is another one of the six breaths, where it indicates a blowing form of exhalation, performed with rounded lips.

Next, the *Zhuangzi* speaks of "blowing out the old and drawing in the new" (*tugu naxin* 吐故納新). The word *tu*, "to blow out" or "to spit," implies that the breath was exhaled through the mouth, while *na*, "to draw in," is written with the "silk" radical and suggests a subtle drawing in from the outside. The expression also indicates the vision of *qi* as breath in ancient China, i.e., the concept that by exchanging oxygen and carbon dioxide in the body new energy is brought into the system and old remnants are released. This is expressed in some more detail in a fragment of the *Yangsheng yaoji* 養生要集 (Essential

Compendium on Nourishing Life), a medieval work in ten sections that was lost in the Tang dynasty.[3] The text says:

> Liu Jun'an says:[4] Eating live *qi* and blowing out dead *qi* you can live long. That is to say, as you draw the *qi* in through the nose it is alive; as you blow it out through the mouth it is dead. Ordinary folk cannot absorb *qi*, since to do so one must make constant efforts from morning to night and only then can one gradually extend the ingestion of *qi*. Without interruption one must draw it in through the nose and blow it out through the mouth. That is what we call "blowing out the old and drawing in the new." (Stein 1999, 174)

Respiration, also expressed generally with the term *xi* 息, which indicates the resting period between the rhythmic rising and falling of the breath in analogy to the alternation of yin and yang, is therefore a major means for the constant exchange of new and old energies in the body, a way to regulate the balance between inner and outer, and a method to regulate the various vital energies in the human body.

According to Chinese medical theory, the main organ involved in breathing is the lungs, where the heavenly *qi*—air, sunlight, cosmic energies—first enters the body and is transformed into ancestral *qi* (*zongqi* 宗氣). From here the ancestral *qi* moves down into the kidneys, where it is mixed with inherent, original or primordial *qi* (*yuanqi* 元氣) to bring forth perfect *qi* (*zhenqi* 真氣).

The latter is what keeps the person alive by circulating through all the organs and is therefore a key factor in cultivation practice. It is important that the perfect *qi* remains pure, which means that all forms of stale or used *qi* need to be eliminated from the body. This happens primarily through exhalation—again the task of the lungs (Engelhardt 1996,18). The lungs, at the borderline between the inner body and the outside world, thus occupy a key position and are considered the protective canopy of all the organs. The six healing breaths are therefore part of the cleansing and purifying of the body, essential for the maintenance of a smooth and harmonious energetic exchange.

---

[3] The work is attributed to the *Liezi* 列子 commentator Zhang Zhan 張湛 of the fourth century. See Sakade 1986a; Despeux 1989; Stein 1999.

[4] Liu Jun'an 劉君安 is Liu Gen 劉根, a famous immortal of the Later Han dynasty. A hermit on Mount Song, he used various longevity techniques and acquired the ability to raise the dead. See DeWoskin 1983, 82-83; Campany 2002, 240-48.

The Six Breaths

The technique of the six breaths follows the ancient vision of "blowing out the old and drawing in the new," i.e., it proposes inhalation through the nose and exhalation through the mouth. Each breath is associated with a particular character, defined in some detail in ancient dictionaries, notably the *Shuowen jiezi zhu* 說文解字注 (Annotated Character Explanation) of the Han dynasty and the *Kangxi zidian* 康熙字典 (Kangxi Dictionary) of the eighteenth century. They are:

> 1. Si 呬四 is a gentle, relaxed exhalation that lets the breath escape between slightly opened lips.
>
> 2. He 呵 or xu 呴 is a strong breath with open mouth that is accompanied by a guttural rasping through tightening of the throat at the base of the tongue. Also described as a hot breath, it may serve to expel burning or heat.
>
> 3. Hu 呼, the standard term for "exhale," indicates a blowing out of breath with rounded lips.
>
> 4. Xu 噓 is a gentle expulsion of breath. The mouth is wide open and the air is released from the bottom of the lungs. When placing a hand in front of the mouth, one gets a feeling of lukewarm air
>
> 5. Chui 吹 indicates a sharp expulsion of air, with lips almost closed and the mouth barely open. It is a puffing out of air that creates the feeling of a cold draft.
>
> 6. Xi 嘻 / 唏 is traditionally the sound of sighing. It describes a soft exhalation with the mouth slightly open that comes deep from within the body (see Maspero 1981, 497-98).

Among the six, the most complex is the second, *he* or *xu*. The word *he* in the *Kangxi Dictionary* is associated with various oral noises, including angry grunts, laughter, and belching (*Chou*, 7a). *Xu*, on the other hand is the older of the two, already in the *Zhuangzi* joined with *chui* to form the compound "huff and puff." The same pair also appears in the Mawangdui 馬王堆 (Hunan) manuscript *Quegu shiqi* 卻穀食氣 (Abstaining from Grains and Eating *Qi*), which was buried in 168 B.C.E. and unearthed in 1973. The text deals with techniques of eliminating grains and ordinary foodstuffs from the diet and replacing them with medicinal herbs and *qi* through special breathing exercises which will free the body from stale and pathogenic *qi* (Ma 1992, 829; Harper 1998, 130). It repeatedly contrasts "those who eat *qi*" with "those who eat grain" and states: "Who eats *qi* should regularly exhale *xu* and *chui* whenever one lies down or gets up" (Engelhardt 2001, 220). Its thrust is also recouped in the *Lunheng* 論衡 (Balanced Discussions) of the second century C.E., which says: "Those who live on *qi* must in all cases practice the techniques of inhaling and exhaling, huffing and puffing, blowing out the old and drawing in the new" (ch. 24; see Sakade 1986c, 8).

Another early mention of these healing breaths appears in the *Yinshu* 引書 (Stretch Book), a text found among medical manuscripts at Zhangjiashan 張家山 (Hunan) in 1984 and dated to 186 B.C.E. (Wenwu 1990). The text includes over a hundred instructions and presents three major kinds of breathing exercises—inhaling the pure *qi* of Heaven and Earth; holding the breath; and exhaling with *chui*, *xu*, and *hu*. The latter represent fine, subtle, and sharp exhalation respectively. They are practiced differently according to the seasons:

> Lie down on your back and exhale with *chui* and *xu* in order to pull in yin-[*qi*]. In spring, exhale several times with *xu* plus once each with *hu* and *chui*. In summer, exhale several times with *hu* plus once each with *xu* and *chui*. In [fall and] winter, exhale several times with *chui* plus once each with *xu* and *hu*. (Wenwu 1990, 86; Engelhardt 2001, 220)

The effect of this method includes the control of excessive emotions as well the expulsion of harmful influences from the body, such as dryness (*hu*), dampness (*chui*), and heat (*xu*).

A pictural illustration of some exhalation methods, notably *hu*, is also found in another early manuscript, the *Daoyin tu* 導引圖 (Healing Exercise Chart), discovered in Mawangdui (see Harper 1998, 310-27; Leong 2001). Consisting of forty-four depictions of men and women practicing various exercise moves—for the most part standing, but also some in seated positions—the chart has three instances where breathing appears prominently. Illustrations number 25, 34, and 35 all show standing figures with arms raised above the head or held near the belly and mouths open. Their captions in each case indicate that the person is making a sound, either "calling [like a crane]" (#25), "exhaling [while raising the head]" (# 34), or "shouting [like a monkey to dispel heat]" (#35) (Harper 1998, 315). The word for "exhale," moreover, seems to be a character variant of *hu*.

In addition to the manuscript sources, there are several more main-stream occurrences of "huff and puff" in ancient texts, most notably in the *Daode jing* 道德經 (Book of the Dao and Its Virtue). The text says:

> Whoever wants to control the world with intentional action
> I know cannot succeed.
> The world is a divine vessel that cannot be run with inten-
> tion.
> Intentional action means defeat,
> Tight control is the beginning of loss.
> Thus among all beings,
> Some lead and some follow,
> Some puff (*xu*) and some huff (*chui*),
> Some are strong, some feeble,
> Some are calm, some agitated.
> For this reason, the sage eliminates all excess, all flourishes,
> and all luxury. (ch. 29)

Most commentators do not pay particular attention to "puff and huff." Among those who do, some associate *xu* with weaker or feebler crea-tures and take *chui* to indicate the stronger and more forceful ones. Another reading is that *xu* indicates a breath that will warm the body, while *chui* is a technique of cooling. For example, the Later Han com-mentator Heshang gong 河上公 or Master on the River (see Chan 1991) states that "*xu* recreates warmth, *chui* recovers cool" (ch. 29). The *Xiang'er zhu* 想爾注 (Xiang'er Commentary), dated to around 200, notes the same thing, then continues: "The good and the bad follow the same rule, health and sickness have the same root" (Rao 1992, 39).[5] This division into hot and cold, moreover, matches not only the *Yinshu* of old, but also notes found in the Tang commentary to the *Zhuangzi*, where Cheng Xuanying 成玄英 suggests that *xu* is a heated breath that opens the body for the reception of new *qi*, while *chui* is a cool breath that relieves symptoms of cold and the expulsion of the stale (ch. 15).

By the mid-Tang, the association of *xu* with heat was firmly estab-lished and the character was even written with the "fire" radical. Also, at this time the variant *he* first appears. Thus, the *Taiqing diaoqi jing* 太清調氣經 (Great Clarity Scripture on Harmonizing *Qi*, DZ 820) of the eighth century uses the word *he*, which it treats as synonymous

---

[5] For more on the concepts of health and personal cultivation in the *Xiang'er Commentary*, including also a full translation, see Bokenkamp 1997.

with *tu* and describes as the blowing out of hot pathogenic energies.[6]
The text says:

> Whether walking, standing, sitting, or lying down, always
> inhale through the nose and exhale (*hetu*) through the
> mouth. Inhaling you draw in the pure [*qi*], exhaling you ex-
> pel the stale [*qi*]. It is stale because it comes from the five
> inner organs. Why is it that the five organs have stale *qi*? It
> is because of eating the five flavors. Each of the five flavors
> corresponds to one of the organs, and each organ's stale *qi* is
> eliminated through the mouth. . . .
>
> In all cases when the inside of the mouth is dry and the in-
> ner skin of the jaws feels rough and without saliva, or again
> if there is pain in the throat and one is unable to eat, this
> indicates a condition of heat. To alleviate it, open the mouth
> wide and exhale with *he*. With each *he*, use the proper gate
> [nose] and window [mouth]. Repeat ten or twenty times.
> (5ab; Huang and Wurmbrand 1987, 1:74)

Here the medical therapeutics of breathing are made clear, with *he* or
xu an effective way to relieve excess heat and dryness in the body.[7]
Another mid-Tang note on this breath is found in Sun Simiao's 孫思邈
Qianjin yaofang 千金要方 (Essential Prescriptions Worth a Thousand
Gold Pieces), dated to 652 and nowadays conveniently available in a
punctuated edition (Sun 1992).

Sun states that *xu* is the name of the body god who resides in the
heart (ch. 13). Although none of the other deities have names even
remotely linked to the six breaths, this allows the speculation that
the six breaths in Daoism may have been closely related to the invo-
cation of body divinities. This understanding is substantiated by the
denial of just such a relationship. The ninth-century *Huangting neijing wuzang liufu buxie tu* 黃庭內景五臟六腑補瀉圖 (Illustrated Manual on the Tonification and Dispersal [of Qi] in the Five Organs and

---

6 Another eighth-century work still uses *xu*. See *Yanling xiansheng ji
xinjiu fuqi jing* 延陵先生集新舊服氣經 (Master Yanling's Scripture of Collected
Old and New Methods of *Qi*-Absorption, DZ 825). A partial translation is
found in Maspero 1981, 476-79.

7 This notion is also reflected in the *Lingjianzi* 靈劍子 (Master of the
Numinous Sword, DZ 570; trl. Huang and Wurmbrand 1987, 2:45-74) of the
mid-Tang which emphasizes that there is no need to use all six breaths but
that *xu* and *chui* will be perfectly sufficient since they eliminate the main
causes of disease. See Ding 1993, 19.

Six Viscera According to the Inner Yellow Court Scripture, DZ 432),[8] hereafter called *Buxie tu* says: "The six characters [for the six breaths] describe the *qi* of the inner organs. They are not the names of deities. Those who make use of the six breaths need to know that they are exclusively used for the expulsion of diseases and must not be confused with embryo respiration" (21b). This makes it clear that the main focus of the practice of the six breaths in medieval China was medical and restorative rather than meditative and geared toward immortality. Within this framework, moreover, there were three major theories that each linked the breaths with the organs in a particular way.

Master Daolin's Method

The first theory regarding the six healing breaths is found in chapter 27 of Sun Simiao's *Qianjin yaofang* under the heading "Longevity Methods of Master Daolin." Daolin has been identified as Zhi Daolin 支道林 or Zhi Dun 支沌 (314-366), an early aristocratic Buddhist and possibly one of the compilers of the *Yangsheng yaoji* (Sakade 1986b, 68; Barrett 1982, 41).

His method also appears in a separate text in the Daoist canon: the *Taiqing Daolin shesheng lun* 太清道林儔生論 (Great Clarity Discourse on Protecting Life by Master Daolin, DZ 1427), hereafter abbreviated *Daolin lun*. A short text of twenty-four pages, this describes different prescriptions and prohibitions regarding life style, living quarters, and diet. It also outlines massages, exercises, and breathing techniques. Although this text does not show in bibliographies until the Song, the fact that it is closely identical with passages in Sun Simiao's work and associated with the *Yangsheng yaoji* makes a pre-Tang date likely (see Despeux 1989).

This supposition is further supported by the fact that Master Daolin's method of breathing is also summarized in the *Zhubing yuanhou lun* 諸病源侯論 (The Origins and Symptoms of Medical Disorders), a major medical encyclopedia compiled by a group of imperially appointed physicians under the guidance of Chao Yuanfang 巢元方 in 610 (see

---

[8] The text is ascribed to the Daoist nun Hu An 胡愔, who lived on Mount Taibai and was also known as the Master of Manifesting Simplicity (Jiansuzi 見素子). It has a preface dated to 848. See Needham 1983, 82.

Despeux and Obringer 1997). Arranged according to symptoms, this work is unique in that it provides both medical and herbal methods according to the traditional medical model alongside various longevity techniques, including exercises, breathing, diets, and others. The six healing breaths feature prominently in the chapter on the ailments of the five inner organs (ch. 15; Ding 1993, 18).

Another albeit abbreviated version of the same early system is also found in the *Yangxing yanming lu* 養性延命錄 (On Nourishing Inner Nature and Extending Life, DZ 838) ascribed to either Tao Hongjing 陶弘景 (456-536) or Sun Simiao and closely echoing the *Yangsheng yaoji*.[9] The text consists of six sections: General Principles, Dietetics, Prohibitions, *Qi* Absorption, Massages and Healing Exercises, and Alchemical Practices. It describes the six breaths under "Qi Absorption":

> To circulate the *qi*, inhale through the nose and exhale through the mouth. Allow the breath to become subtle and draw it out longer. This is called the long breath. Its inhalation is just one, but its exhalation comes in six different forms. The one way to inhale is with the sound of *xi*, the six ways to exhale involve the sounds *chui, hu, xi, he, xu,* and *si*. Ordinary people breathe one *xi*, one *hu*, and originally that was all.
>
> If you want to practice the exhalation method of the long breath, use *chui* when you are cold and *hu* when you are warm. The breaths are most excellent in curing diseases. *Chui* will drive out wind; *hu* will drive out heat; *xi* will drive out afflictions; *he* will make the *qi* descend; *xu* will disperse blockages; and *si* will moderate extremes [stress]. Since ordinary people are frequently given to extremes, they will use a lot of *xu* and *si. Xu* and *si* are the core of the long breath. (2.2b-3a; Ding 1993, 16)[10]

---

[9] The text is also partly contained in *Yunji qiqian* 32. The *Yunji qiqian* 雲笈七籤 (Seven Tablets in a Cloudy Satchel, DZ 1032) is an encyclopedia of Daoist materials from the early Song dynasty, dated to 1023. A concordance to the text is found in Schipper 1980. Unlike most other authors (Switkin 1987; Mugitani 1987; Despeux 1989), Maspero dates it to the Song, between 1013 when Laozi received the title Hunyuan 混元 (which is used in the text) and 1161 when the *Tongzhi* 通志 (Pervasive Record) lists it (1981, 485n78).

[10] The therapeutic classification of the breaths, in contrast to that using the organ system, is first found in a fourth-century work, the *Shenxian shiqi jin'gui miaolu* 神仙食氣金櫃妙錄 (Wondrous Record of the Golden Casket on the Divine Immortals' Practice of Eating *Qi*, DZ 836, 5b). After that, it also

This emphasizes the medical importance of the practice. More specifically, in a later section, the text notes:

> People with heart disease tend to have cold and heat in their bodies which can be eliminated by using the two breaths *hu* and *chui*, while people with lung problems often feel distension and fullness in their chest and back which the *xu* breath will cure. Also, people with spleen diseases tend to have an upward floating wind and a habitual itchy ache in their bodies which the *xi* breath will eliminate, while people with liver ailments often suffer from eye pain, worry, anxiety, and no joy which is helped by the *he* breath. (4a)

Unlike this fairly technical, medical way of dealing with the six breaths, the *Taishang Laojun yangsheng jue* 太上老君養生訣 (Lord Lao's Formula on Nourishing Life, DZ 821) of the ninth century focuses on its more spiritual dimension.[11] In the context of providing instructions for several physical practices, it describes two different theories on how the six breaths relate to the inner organs.[12] Finding cosmic energy in human breath, it notes that the Ocean of *Qi* (the lower elixir field in the abdomen) collects cosmic power "just as mountains gather clouds and the earth gathers marshes" (5a). Adepts should exercise both in the morning and at night, breathing deeply and consciously and repeating the exercise ten times. The section ends with a renewed emphasis on the human body as constituted by spirit and *qi* and the need to cultivate both in order to attain the Dao (Kohn 1998, 80-81). The text shows that in the ninth century two competing theories of the six breaths were current and that Daoists made use of both to their best advantage.

As used in all these sources, Master Daolin's method of breathing links the six breaths with the inner organs. It says:

> If you suffer from a cold condition of the heart, exhale using *hu*. In case of heart heat, blow out *chui*. For ailments of the

---

appears, with a minor variation, in the *Yanling fuqi jing* (DZ 825, 21b) and the *Huanzhen xiansheng fu neiqi juefa* 幻真先生服內氣訣法 (Master Huanzhen's Essential Method of Absorbing Internal *Qi*, DZ 828). See Maspero 1981, 469; Ding 1993, 18.

[11] On the text, see Ren and Zhong 1991, 587; Kohn 1998, 80-81; Maspero 1981, 463.

[12] It outlines the first theory (Daolin's method) on pp. 5b-7b and the second (*Daoyin jing*) on pp. 2ab.

liver, the breath is *xu*; for those of the lungs, it is *he*. To cure problems of the spleen, exhale with the *xi* breath; for those of the kidneys, use *si*. (*Qianjin yaofang* 27; Sun 1992, 483)[13]

The text continues to specify the numbers of exhalations to be undertaken at certain times of day. It says:

At the midnight hour (11 p.m.-1 a.m.), practice 81 expulsions of breath. At cockcrow (1-3 a.m.), practice 72. At first light (3-5 a.m.), do 63; at sunrise (5-7 a.m.), perform 54. Around the time of breakfast (7-9 a.m.), it is best to breathe out 45 times, while in mid-morning (9-11 a.m.), one should expel the breath 36 times.[14]

Before undertaking the method, it is furthermore best to first stretch and [mentally] guide the *qi* to the right and left [sides of the body] 360 times.[15] The method serves to cure all four basic kinds of ailments: diseases caused by contaminations, restrictions due to cold, illnesses because of wind, and the toxic influxes of heat.[16]

As people suffering from any of these ailments calm their spirits and harmonize their breath, they can be assured of a cure. Each of the five inner organs is subject to 81 diseases caused by cold, heat, wind, or *qi* [contamination]. That makes a total of 404 ailments.[17] In each case, one must know the disease category as defined by the symptoms. (ch. 27; Sun 1992, 483)

The close correlation of the breaths with specific hours can be related to methods of exorcism as part of healing, which goes back to the understanding of illness in ancient China as caused by the invasion ei-

---

[13] The same passage is also found in the *Daolin jing* (DZ 821, 19a); however, it reverses the breaths for the liver and the lungs.

[14] The *Daoyin jing* has somewhat lower numbers, beginning with twenty-four and moving down by a count of six (19b).

[15] The *Daoyin jing* here specifies that practitioners should first undertake the eighteen gymnastic postures and twenty-four self-massages (19b).

[16] These correspond to the basic causes of disease in Chinese medicine as also described in the *Zhubing yuanhou lun*, which moreover explains that contaminations are pathological factors that enter into the body and then stay there, obstructing the *qi* and causing all sorts of problems and imbalances (ch. 24).

[17] The math is off here. It should be 405. The number 404 is more common in Buddhist sources, where 101 ailments are known for each element: water, fire, earth, and air.

ther of noxious *qi* or by demons (Unschuld 1985, 20). This notion was particularly common among early organized Daoist groups who eschewed all medical intervention in favor of confessions, prayers, and petitions to the gods (see Tsuchiya 2002).

Demon medicine survived also in the later medical tradition. Thus Sun Simiao, in the *Qianjin yifang* 千金翼方 (Supplementary Prescriptions Worth a Thousand Gold Pieces), lists the six healing breaths as one of six methods of exorcism or "prohibition" (*jin* 禁), including clicking the teeth, guarding the eyes, chasing illness with thought, sacred gestures, and visualization of body gods (ch. 29; Sun 1983). In all cases, the methods should be undertaken in the proper alignment with yin and yang, the falling and rising of living *qi* in the course of the day. The times given for the six breaths are all in the yang period of the day, between midnight and noon, providing an optimal chance for healing by relating the practitioner to living, rising *qi*.

Moving on from this, Sun next lists the specific symptoms for the five inner organs. He begins with the heart, whose ailments can be recognized by symptoms related to the corresponding phase. People with heart-based conditions, for example, will be terrified of fire in their dreams. Also, the color that goes with the heart is red, and accordingly patients will dream of people dressed in red or of those holding a red baton or saber. The breath to use is *hu* when there is excess cold and *chui* for excess heat. It is best to practice the exhalation for thirty (cold) or fifty (heat) forceful repetitions, followed by ten subtle ones.

The breaths for the organs are:

organ	phase	color	symptoms	*qi*	reps
heart	fire	red	excess heat/cold, fire in dreams, red batons, cold	*hu*	30/10
			heat	*chui*	50/10
liver	wood	green	melancholy, eye trouble, green dreams, tigers, wolves	*he*	30/10
spleen	earth	yellow	aches, yellow in dreams, infants playing with dangers	*xi*	30/10
lungs	metal	white	swellings, dream of charming people, family members	*xu*	30/10
kidney	water	black	excess cold, dream of terrifying animals, often black	*si*	50/10

The method is to be used patiently and consistently, and with an attitude of humility and reverence. It is certain to cure all sorts of ailments and to restore health and balance to the inner organs.

Master Ning's Model

Also going back to medieval China, another early model of the six breaths uses a completely different alignment with the inner organs and, instead of having two different breaths for the heart, it adds the Triple Heater as a sixth organ. The Triple Heater (*sanjiao* 三焦), sometimes also called the Triple Burner, is a uniquely Chinese organ. Described in the early texts on Chinese medicine, it provides a connection between Heaven (upper heater), Humanity (middle heater), and Earth (lower heater). Over time these three sections came to be associated with three aspects of the body cavity: thoracic, abdominal, and pelvic, i.e., the lungs, small intestine, and bladder. Commencing its function immediately after birth, the Triple Heater system serves to control the transport, utilization, and excretion of the body's energies.

The model that first introduces the Triple Heater into the six breaths is found in the *Taiqing daoyin yangsheng jing* 太清導引養生經 (Great Clarity Scripture of Healing Exercises and Nourishing Life, DZ 818), [18] hereafter abbreviated *Daoyin jing*, which contains a wide range of information about different Daoist schools of healing exercises. Although not mentioned in bibliographies until 1145, it is based on sources that go back to the sixth century or earlier and has many fragments and quotations both in Daoist and in medical literature. The text may also be a fragment of the *Yangsheng yaoji*, which was only lost in the eighth century and may have surfaced again in the Song under the title *Daoyin jing* (Despeux 1989, 229-30).

The six breaths are described in the chapter on the "Healing Exercises of Master Ning" and are called a technique of "exercises and *qi* awareness" (*daoyin siqi* 導引思氣). Master Ning 寧先生 is a semi-legendary immortal of old who, according to the *Liexian zhuan* 列仙傳 (Immortals' Biographies, DZ 294) of the Han dynasty, lived in the era of the Yellow Emperor and excelled in various body exercises (Kaltenmark 1953, 43-47). He patterned his practice on animal imitations,

---

[18] The text also occurs in an abbreviated format in *Yunji qiqian* 34 and *Daoshu* 28. On the *Yunji qiqian*, see note 11 above. The *Daoshu* 道樞 (Pivot of the Dao, DZ 1017) is a collection of self-cultivation and inner alchemical methods by Zeng Zao 曾慥 (d.1151). For a study, see Miyazawa 1984. A detailed discussion and translation is found in Kohn, forthcoming.

including the toad, tortoise, and dragon—creatures associated my-
thologically with the moon and with various bodies of water.[19]

His model of the six breaths also appears in five other Tang-dynasty
Daoist texts, including the *Taiqing diaoqi jing* mentioned earlier.[20]
They all discuss the absorption, circulation, and refinement of *qi* as
well as methods of visualization and embryo respiration. The same
model, moreover, also appears in a Buddhist text, the *Xiuxi zhiguan
zuochan fayao* 修習止觀坐禪法要 (Essential Methods of Cultivating
Concentration, Insight, and Absorption, T. 1915, 46.462-475)[21] by
Zhiyi 智顗 (538-597), the founder of the Tiantai 天台 school. If this
ascription is correct, this text would contain the earliest clearly dat-
able description of this model, however, the style of the passage in
seven-character verse suggests a later, maybe even Song-dynasty,
insertion. The text says:

> It is sufficient to devote oneself to insight practice by con-
> centrating one's spirit on the six kinds of breath. As one
> learns to use the six breaths one can heal diseases and pur-
> sue insight more easily. What are the six breaths? They are
> *chui, hu, he, xu, si,* and *xi.* These six kinds of respiration are
> thought of mentally as one first moves the breath in the
> mouth, then when it has been well revolved exhales it very
> softly. The relevant poem runs:
>
> The heart corresponds to *he* [*hu/chui*]; the kidneys match
> *chui* [*si*];[22]
> The spleen is *hu* [*xi*]; the lungs relate to *si* [*he*]—

---

[19] A text specifically associated with Master Ning was lost but survives
in citations in the *Yangsheng yaoji* as found in Tamba no Yasuyori's 丹波康瀬
Ishimpō 醫心方 (Essential Medical Methods), a Japanese medical encyclopedia dated to 984 (27.22a).

[20] The other four are the *Taishang laojun yangsheng jue* (see above, note
13); the *Taiwu xiansheng fuqi fa* 太無先生服氣法 (Master Great Nonbeing's
Method of *Qi* Absorption, DZ 824, also *Yunji qiqian* 59), probably of the late
eighth century (Maspero 1981, 460-61, 507); the *Huanzhen juefa* (DZ 828,
also *Yunji qiqian* 60.14a-25b), a text of the mid-Tang (Maspero 1981, 461);
and the *Taixi biyao gejue* 胎息秘要歌訣 (Song and Formula of the Secret Es-
sentials of Embryo Respiration, DZ 131, trl. Huang and Wurmbrand 1987,
1:43-48).

[21] The abbreviation T. stands for *Taishō Daizōkyō* 大正大藏經, the Japanese edition of the Buddhist canon. The numbers refer to text, volume, and
page.

[22] Words in brackets indicate the breaths according to Master Daolin's
Method to show the degree of difference.

All the sages know this.
When the liver is subject to heat, it can be treated with *xu*
[*he*].
When the Triple Heater is obstructed, work with *xi*. (471c-
72a)

In the *Daoyin jing*, the breaths are listed in a slightly different order
and further elaborated in terms of body correspondences and specific
conditions to be treated. For example, the first breath is *he*:

> In the practice of exercises and *qi* awareness, *he* belongs to
> the heart which governs the tongue. All conditions of dry-
> ness in the mouth and obstruction of *qi* as well as of bad
> breath can be cured by breathing *he*. If you are very hot,
> open the mouth wide; if you are a little hot, open the mouth
> a little. Be conscious about how many breaths you need to
> affect a cure and lessen repetitions as you go along. (16a)

Similarly, *hu* is related to the spleen and helps with conditions of low
fever and discomfort, a feeling of fullness in belly, stomach, and intestines, bad circulation, and energetic compression. Third, *xu* belongs to
the liver which governs the eyes; it is effective in cases of inflamed
and congested eyes and other vision troubles. The next breath is *chui*,
which corresponds to the kidneys and the ears and helps in cases of
abdominal cold, infertility, and hearing afflictions. Fifth comes *si*, the
breath of the lungs and the nose, very effective in cases of tempera-
ture imbalances and skin troubles. Sixth and finally—not mentioned
in the *Daoyin jing*, but supplied in the other texts—the *xi* breath activates the Triple Heater and alleviates all maladies associated with
this digestive and energy-processing organ (16ab). The *Daoyin jing*
concludes by saying:

> Each of the six breaths—*he*, *si*, *hu*, *xu*, *chui*, and *xi*—is
> ruled by one of the five organs. In case of extreme fatigue,
> one can use them easily to regulate the *qi* and improve one's
> condition.

Master Ning's model of the six breaths can be described as a detailed
medical way of treating various imbalances of *qi* associated with the
five inner organs and the Triple Heater. It follows the standard correspondence system of Chinese medicine, is both therapeutic and preventative, and can address a large number of different conditions.
Using the various versions of the list in the different Daoist texts we
find the following symptoms for the breaths:

heart	*he*	oral dryness and roughness, *qi* obstructions, pathogenic *qi*, heat, heart conditions, emotional states
liver	*xu*	inflamed, teary, or red eyes; liver conditions; vision problems; rising *qi*
spleen	*hu*	fast and hot *qi*, abdominal swelling, *qi* obstruction, dry lips, spleen conditions, arm and leg issues
lungs	*si*	temperature imbalance, lung problems, abscesses, skin issues, nasal obstructions, fatigue, exhaustion, oppression
kidneys	*chui*	coldness in the back and joints, genital problems, deafness, ear conditions
heater	*xi*	all conditions associated with the Triple Heater

The model is different from the earlier method in that it shows a more rational approach to disease and leaves out the various dream symptoms, but it also has less detail in terms of times and numbers of repetitions. Beyond that, and despite its reduction of the heart to a single breath, it still retains the previous emphasis on this organ. It says:

> Although each of these breaths will cure ailments, neverthe-less the five organs and the Triple Heater as well as all symptoms of cold, heat, fatigue, bad breath, and other dis-eases are all related to the heart. Since the heart matches the *he* breath, using this breath can cure all manner of ail-ments. It is not necessary to employ all six. (7b-8a; Maspero 1981, 497)

This suggests that the importance of the heart continued in the tradi-tion of the six breaths even as the matching of correspondences changed, the Triple Heater was added as a sixth organ, and the medi-cal symptoms became more detailed and less dream-centered.

Master Ning's model of the six breaths was later codified in various longevity collections and is still the standard today. It first appears in the *Xiuzhen shishu* 修真十書 (Ten Works on the Cultivation of Perfec-tion; DZ 263) of the year 1131, an extensive compilation in sixty scrolls of inner alchemical and body cultivation methods (see Maspero 1981, 515). Here the six breaths appear in the order *chui* (kidneys), *he* (heart), *xu* (liver), *si* (lungs), *hu* (spleen), and *xi* (Triple Heater), right after a seated exercise sequence known as the "Eight Brocades." A poem appended to their general description and ascribed to Sun Simiao, moreover, associates the breaths with the four seasons:

> In spring, breathe *xu* for clear eyes and so wood can aid
> your liver.
> In summer, reach for *he* so heart and fire are at peace.

> In fall, breathe *si* to stabilize and gather metal, keeping the
> lungs moist.
> For the kidneys, next, breathe *chui* and see your inner wa-
> ter calm.
>
> The Triple Heater needs your *xi* to expel all heat and trou-
> bles.
> In all four seasons take long breaths, so the spleen can
> process food.
> And, of course, avoid exhaling noisily, not letting even your
> ears hear it.
> This practice is most excellent and will preserve your divine
> elixir. (19.7a; Sakade 1986c, 15)

That the practice was actually undertaken in the Song dynasty, and
not only by Daoists or specialized longevity seekers, is documented in
the *Yijian zhi* 夷堅志 (Record of Wondrous Marvels) by Hong Mai 洪邁
(1123-1202) of twelfth century. The text collects anecdotes of extraordinary events or usual occurrences thought worthwhile by its author.
In chapter 9, it describes the practice of a certain Li Siju 李似矩 who
tended to get up each day at midnight to expel his breath with *xu* and
chui and perform a series of self-massages (Sakade 1986c, 16).

In the Ming dynasty, the six breaths appear in two collections. The
first is the *Huoren xinfa* 活人心法 (Essential Methods for Living People), by the imperial prince Zhu Quan 朱權 (1378-1448), the seventeenth son of the dynasty's founder Zhu Yuanzhang 朱元璋. Also
known as the Hermit of the Great Ming (Da Ming qishi 大明奇士), he
stayed out of politics and spent his time studying, playing the lute,
cultivating flowers, growing bamboo, and pursuing an interest in long
life, medicine, and chemistry. He wrote over fifty books; some on Daoist and literary subjects, and many that discuss healing exercises and
other cultivation methods (DeBryun 2000, 605). The *Huoren xinfa* is
one of his main works on longevity practices; like the *Xiuzhen shishu*,
it presents a description of the six breaths after an illustrated account
of the Eight Pieces of Brocade.

This arrangement is reversed in the other Ming-dynasty description
of the six breaths in the *Chifeng sui* 赤鳳髓 (Marrow of the Red Phoenix; trl. Despeux 1988), a comprehensive outline of physical techniques by Zhou Lüjing 周籚靖 of the year 1578. Here the six breaths,
in the order *he*, *chui*, *xu*, *si*, *hu*, and *xi* are presented after a general
discussion of the principles of *qi* in relation to the four seasons and
before the various exercise patterns, such as the Five Animals' Frolic,

the Eight Pieces of Brocade, and a series of forty-six moves associated
with various immortals. The breaths are introduced with a general
formula that involves a specific body posture for each organ. It says:

> The liver: as you exhale with *xu*, make sure the eyes are
> wide open.
> The lungs: as you exhale with *si*, make sure the two hands
> protect the lungs.
> The heart: the *he* breath corresponds to the heart; cross the
> two hands above the head.
> *Chui*: this matches the kidneys; wrap your arms around the
> knees.
> For spleen symptoms: as you exhale with *hu*, best pucker
> the mouth.
> If heat enters the Triple Heater, do not be concerned;
> The immortals' breath *xi* is a subtle and powerful secret.
> Practice these six daily and your body will feel ever better.
>   (ch. 6; Despeux 1988, 98)

As for the breaths themselves, the text includes cosmic correspondences, such as pointing out that the liver is connected with the green
dragon, the east, and spring, as well as specific symptoms of the organ in question which can be alleviated by the practice. All in all, the
account here closely matches the medieval system, showing that Master Ning's model has remained dominant over the centuries.

The Yellow Court Version

Some aspects of Master Ning's model further developed in a yet different variant of the system associated with three Tang-dynasty texts
written in the tradition of the *Huangting jing* 黃庭經 (Yellow Court
Scripture, DZ 403), a work in multiple parts that goes back to the
early Highest Clarity (Shangqing 上清) school of the fourth century
and is characterized by extensive body visualizations and meditative
focus on the five inner organs.[23] The Yellow Court version uses the
same correspondences of breaths to organs but with two differences:
it replaces the Triple Heater with the gall bladder as a sixth organ;
and it assigns dispersing (cooling) and tonifying (heating) properties
to each of the breaths.

---

[23] For discussions of the text, see Maspero 1981; Robinet 1993.. Partial
translations appear in Homann 1971; Kroll 1996. For a punctuated edition
and index, see Schipper 1975.

For example, the *Taishang yangsheng taixi qi jing* 太上養生胎息經 (Great Scripture on Nourishing Life Through Embryo Respiration and *Qi*, DZ 819) of the Tang dynasty, hereafter abbreviated *Taixi jing*, begins with the note that by following the teachings of the *Daode jing*, the *Huangting jing*, and the *Yangsheng yaoji* one can eliminate all ten thousand diseases (5b). It then characterizes each breath in a seven-word verse and specifies that it can be used either to disperse or to tonify *qi*. Applying the productive sequence of the five phases in the so-called mother-child system, each breath disperses or cools the *qi* in the preceding organ and tonifies or heats it in the following (5b-7b; see also Ding 1993, 17). That is to say:

phase	organ	cool	heat
wood	liver	*xu*	*chui*
fire	heart	*he*	*xu*
earth	spleen	*hu*	*he*
metal	lungs	*si*	*hu*
water	kidneys	*chui*	*si*
	gallbladder	*xi*	*xu*

The system as presented here is thus a bit more complex than earlier versions in that it takes into account the close interrelation among the inner organs and their productive dynamics. It is not sufficient to just exhale in a certain way to deal with ailments in a specific organ, but one must consider the entire pattern. Beyond this, the text also allows for practice beyond the yang hours between midnight and noon and specifies the ideal numbers of exhalations. It says:

> Practice at midnight [11 p.m.-1 a.m.], 9 x 9 or 81 times.
> Practice at dawn [3-5 a.m.], 8 x 8 or 64 times.
> Practice at breakfast [7-9 a.m.], 7 x 7 or 49 times.
> Practice at noon [11a.m.-1 p.m.], 6 x 6 or 36 times.
> Practice in mid-afternoon [3-5 p.m.], 5 x 5 or 25 times.
> Practice at dusk [7-9 p.m.], 4 x 4 or 16 times. (1ab)

Another text that presents this version is the ninth-century *Buxie tu* (DZ 432). After citing Sun Simiao on a general exposition of the nature of the body, it provides a detailed description of each inner organ plus the gall bladder, including the name and an illustration of the resident body god in the form of a mythical animal (see Fig. 1). It also outlines the relevant symptoms together with specific procedures on how to nourish and maintain organ health as well as diagnostic elements and detailed recipes. Following this, the text specifies which breath to practice, how to activate the organ with the help of healing exercises, and what diet to prefer. To give an example:

Using the *si* breath. Begin with a long, soft inhalation through the nose, followed by a *si* exhalation through the mouth, all without making a sound. Before the practice always harmonize the *qi* to make it flow evenly. Then practice *si*. If the lungs are afflicted by an ailment, use thirty forceful *si* expulsions, followed by thirty subtle ones.

This will eliminate all strain and heat from the lungs, cure all coughs and wheezes due to rising *qi*, and take care of all boils and afflictions of the skin. It is also good for states of fatigue and pain in the limbs, nasal congestion due to cold, and pains in the back and chest. As the healing takes effect, lessen the number of repetitions. (6a)

Similarly, all other sound exercises begin with a long, soft inhalation after having harmonized the *qi* and involve a specific number of expulsions, most commonly thirty forceful and

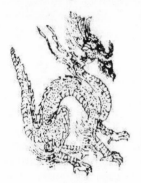

ten subtle ones—as already specified in Daolin's method. Symptoms, again as in the other texts, tend to match medical texts on the various organs and include fatigue and agitation for the heart, vision trouble and rising heat for the liver, cold symptoms and digestive troubles for the spleen, ear troubles and abscesses for the kidneys, and cold conditions and various pains for the gall bladder (12b-21a).

Fig. 1: The liver spirit.

Beyond this general commonality with the other methods, however, the Yellow Court version also has a more ritual and religious dimension. It prescribes that each breathing exercise is executed in meditative posture and accompanied by visualizations that match the breaths with organs, colors, and directions. For example, to tonify the heart, practitioners visualize themselves absorb the red *qi* of the south. In this, the Yellow Court version integrates an ancient Highest Clarity breathing method known as the Five Sprouts" (*wuya* 五芽), which allows adepts to partake of the pure energies of the five directions. Although a way of inhaling rather than exhaling, it is very similar to this version of the six healing breaths in that it connects cosmic regions and colors with the inner organs and allows adepts to cleanse and cosmicize their *qi* with the help of the breath.

To undertake Five Sprouts practice, adepts begin by swallowing saliva while chanting invocations to the original *qi* of the four cardinal directions. Then they face one direction, usually beginning with the east, and visualize the *qi* of that direction in its appropriate color. A general mist in the beginning, it gradually forms into a ball like the rising sun, then through further concentration shrinks in size and is made to approach the adept. Eventually the size of a pill, the Sprout can be swallowed and guided mentally to the organ of its correspondence. A suitable incantation places it firmly in its new receptacle, and gradually the adepts body becomes infused with cosmic energy and partakes more actively of the cosmos as a whole.

The cosmic sprouts, as Isabelle Robinet points out, are originally the "germinal essences of the clouds" or "mist." They represent the yin principle of heaven—that is, the yin within the yang. They manifest in human saliva, again a yin element in the upper, yang, part of the body. They help to nourish and strengthen the five inner organs. The *Daodian lun* 道典論 (On the Code of the Dao, DZ 1130), a Highest Clarity scripture of the fifth century, explains that they are very tender, comparable to the fresh sprouts of plants, and that they assemble at dawn in the celestial capital, from where they spread all over the universe until the sun begins to shine. Turning like the wheels of a carriage, they ascend to the gates of the nine heavens, from where they continue to the medium level of the world—to the five sacred mountains ruled over by the five emperors of the five directions—and finally descend into the individual adept. They thus pass through the three major levels of the cosmos (4.9b-10a; Robinet 1989, 165).

The sprouts contain the potential of being in its nascent state, the imperceptible *qi* in a state of pure becoming. "Sprouting" means inherent creation, purity, newness, return to youth. The practice is accordingly undertaken at dawn, the time when everything awakens to life, yet another symbol of creative, unstructured potential. By ingesting the sprouts, the Daoist partakes of the inherent power of celestial bodies and feeds on the pure creative energy of the universe its most subtle form. It is thus not surprising that the absorption of the sprouts is also used as a preparatory practice for the "abstention from grains." By and by the sprout intake replaces adepts regular nourishment and allows them to identify with the germinal energy of the cosmos. They thus can become lighter and freer, appear and disappear at will, overcome the limitations of this world, and attain immortality in the heavenly realms.

Integrating this early medieval practice with the healing effects of the six breaths, the Yellow Court version joins medical breathing techniques with Daoist practice and allows a broader use of the method. This tendency continued further in the *Shangqing huangting wuzang liufu zhenren yuzhou jing* 上清黃庭五臟六腑真人玉軸經 (Highest Clarity Scripture on the Perfected Person's Jade Technique Regarding the Five Organs and Six Viscera According to the Inner Yellow Court Scripture, DZ 1402), hereafter called *Yuzhou jing*, of the late Tang or early Song dynasty.[24] The text is the first to present the technique of the six breaths in a cosmic, mythological setting. It has the Heavenly Worthy of Primordial Beginning (Yuanshi tianzun 元始天尊), the creator god of the Daoist religion, explain the necessity for health and bodily wholeness to the Yellow Emperor—here as in the medical texts the eternal learner and avid follower of instructions, but also the prospective ideal ruler of the empire. The Heavenly Worthy says:

> How can you find out about the essentials of ruling the people without knowing the arts of controlling the body? If you manage others without properly managing yourself, if you cultivate things on the outside without cultivating the inside—how can you not fail? (1a)

The Yellow Emperor is deeply impressed by these words, kowtows, and humbly asks to be taught the relevant methods. After a general exposition on the nature of human life and body, the Heavenly Worthy discusses the individual organs, like the *Buxie tu* beginning with the lungs. He specifies that the *si* exhalation disperses *qi* while every inhalation tonifies the organ, then sets the lungs into a larger cosmological context (2a). He explains that the lungs belong to the phase metal and are shaped like a hanging chime. Their resident body god looks like a white tiger, controls the person's material soul, and can transform into a jade lad seven inches in height who comes and goes in the body, creating various reactions and emotions (2b). The use of the *si* exhalation not only cures diseases but also calms the body god and has a psychological effect, draining physical obstructions as well as anger and upset. More than that, without the regular practice of *si*, especially in the fall, people will find themselves with declining lung capacity and deteriorating health, making the application of the breath a basic necessity (3a).

---

[24] The text is also found, slightly abridged, in *Yunji qiqian* 14.10a-14a. It is listed under a title that includes the word *daoyin* in a Song bibliography. See Loon 1984, 147. For a summary, see also Ding 1993, 17.

The text continues along the same lines with regard to the other organs, similarly describing their shape, body gods, psychological agent, emotional characteristic, and matching season, as well as insisting on the importance of regular breathing practice. The other organs are (3b-9b):

qi	organ	shape	deity	psych	emotion	season
he	heart	lotus blossom	red bird	spirit	agitation	summer
xu	liver	hanging gourd	green dragon	spirit soul	kindness	spring
hu	spleen	upturned bowl	phoenix	intention	jealousy	late sum
chui	kidney	round rock	white deer	will	obedience	winter
xi	gall	hanging gourd	turtle+ snake		courage	late wint

In each case, the text also describes how the practice will strengthen the psychological agents as the various obstructions are blown out with the appropriate breath and positive virtue begins to arise. The six breaths not only cure diseases but create a more humane awareness as practitioners visualize their gods and integrate the cosmic dimension of the organs into their personal identity.

Modern Forms

The six healing breaths have continued play an important role in Daoist and health practices. Not only linked with times, directions, visualizations, and the enhancement of personal virtue, in the Song dynasty they were also connected to specific body movements.

The *Daoshu* 道樞 (Pivot of the Dao, DZ 1017) by Zeng Zao 曾慥 of the mid-twelfth century uses the same match of breaths and organs but presents them in a different order. The text instructs practitioners to begin by sitting cross-legged and breathing deeply, using the abdominal muscles to enhance respiration, then specifies times, directions, and numbers of repetitions for optimal practice, in each case insisting that the practice be concluded by three swallowings of saliva. The numbers are as follows (35.26a):

midnight	north	3 *he*, 12 *hu*
morning	east	12 *hu*, 7 *si*, 12 *xi*
noon	south	7 *si*, 5 *chui*, 12 *xi*
evening	west	9 *xu*, 3 *he*, 12 *xi*

Following this, Zeng Zao lists a set of simple exercise moves to accompany and enhance the effect of the breaths. They are:

To exhale *xu* [liver], clench the hands into fists and open the
eyes wide and look up.
To exhale *si* [lungs], hold the knees with the hands right
and left, then lift the head.
To exhale *he* [heart], interlace the fingers to embrace the
knees, then lift the head.
To exhale *chui* [kidneys], lie on your back and clench the
hands into fists.
To exhale *hu* [spleen], drop the hands and then place them
to embrace the spleen.
To exhale *xi* [gall bladder], sit up straight and lift the head.
(35.26a; Ding 1993, 18)

These and all previously described aspects of the practice have survived and are still actively undertaken today. Modern adepts use the
same correspondence system that has been dominant since the Tang
dynasty but follow Master Ning's model and use the Triple Heater
rather than the gall bladder as a sixth organ. They also suggest that
some of the sounds should be made while exhaling and others while
inhaling (Ma 1983, 27), employ exhalations methods called *hai*, *hei*,
and *pei*, and have created complete sets of patterns that place the six
breaths into an integrated structure (Miura 1989). Aside from this,
modern adepts provide more scientific, medical reasons for the effectiveness of the breaths, noting that they require a different position-
ing of the lips, tongue, teeth, throat, chest, and abdomen in each case
and thus each have a different impact on the inner organs (Hoshino
1985, 81; Miura 1989).

Among Western practitioners, Mantak Chia in his Healing Tao system makes ample use of the six breaths, calling them the Six Healing
Sounds. Modifying the standard set of breaths slightly (WOOO for
chui), he describes them phonetically in easily understandable letters
rather than transliterations of Chinese and emphasizes both the healing and the spiritual dimensions of the practice. In each case the
emotion of the respective organ is released through the exhalation
and its virtue is encouraged. The practice is closely connected to another basic exercise known as the "Inner Smile." Practitioners dress
comfortably and sit on the edge of a chair, their legs hip-distance
apart, their feet flat on the floor. The back is straight, the head up,
shoulders back and down, chin tucked in slightly. The hands rest
comfortably in the lap, right palm on left. They close or lower the eyes
and breathe normally.

To perform the Inner Smile, they then curve their lips into a slight
smile and expand the smiling feeling along the face, into the neck and

throat, as well as to the thyroid, parathyroid, and thymus glands. Following this, they move the *qi* to the five inner organs, envisioning each with its color, smiling at it, appreciating it for its work, and allowing negative emotions to leave while positive virtues come in. The practice ends with the collection of smiling energy in the lower elixir field, where it is centered by being spiraled first in an outward direction thirty-six times (women counter-clockwise, men clockwise), then twenty-four times in the other direction.

The Six Healing Sounds are a supplementary exercise to the Inner Smile. For example:

> **The Lung Sound.** Place your tongue behind your closed teeth, and with a long, slow exhalation, create the sound SSSS (like the sound of steam coming from a radiator). During each resting period (as you slowly inhale), smile to the lungs. Picture them surrounded by white light and concentrate on [releasing sadness while] feeling the virtue of courage, which is directly related to the lungs' energy. This will help enhance the positive energy of the lungs. (Chia and Chia 1993, 104)

Sometimes, certain movements are added to enhance the practice. In the case of the lungs, the hands are lifted from their resting position on the knees to chest level on the inhalation, then expanded upward in an arch with palms facing the ceiling while the chin is lifted and the head pulled back (Fig. 2). This opens the lung meridian which runs along the inside of the arms. The other organs, sounds, colors, emotions, virtues, and movements are as follows (Chia and Chia 1993, 104-05):

organ	sound	color	emotion	virtue	body movement
lungs	SSSS	white	sadness	righteousness	arms raised overhead, palms up, head back
heart	HAWW	red	agitation	love and joy	arms raised overhead, palms down, head back
liver	SHHH	blue	anger	benevolence	arms raised overhead, palms down, head back
kidney	WOOO	black	fear	wisdom	body bent slightly forward, mind on kidneys
spleen	WHOO	yellow	worry	honesty	hands placed on spleen, fingers pressing
heater	HEEE				body prone, visualizing openness, flow of *qi*

The goal of the practice is to release negative emotional energies and to open both mind and body to a more harmonious *qi*-flow. Followers claim that if practiced daily in conjunction with the Inner Smile it energizes people and makes them more loving towards themselves and kinder towards others. It can also be practiced aiming at specific problems, and should be done more often in times of crisis, stress, anger, fear, or depression.

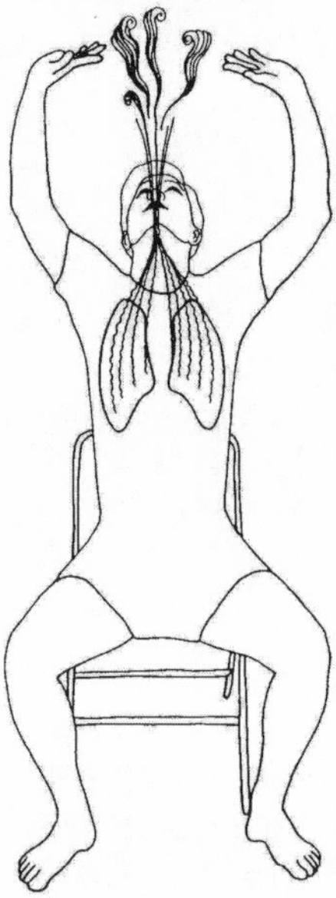

By learning to smile and breathe into the tense part of the body until the tension melts and negative emotions become vital energy, people can learn to express themselves more authentically. Not only healthier and with a greater sense of harmony and well-being, people also find themselves ready to enter the higher stages of Healing Tao practice, which involve the transformation of the self into a divine child and the creation of an inner sense of oneness with the Dao, an empowerment within the body that transcends the limitations of physical existence. The practice of the six healing breaths, originally mostly medical in nature, has thus become a firm part of the spiritual transformation of the individual.

Fig. 2: The Lung Exercise

Conclusion

Breathing is an important aspect of life and plays a key role in spiritual and body cultivation. Although born with the natural ability to breathe slowly and deeply, people commonly are subject to various levels of stress, which causes the breath to become shallow and short. Before long, they accept this as the normal state of affairs and no longer breathe naturally by filling the lungs all the way and stretching the diaphragm so that the abdomen expands upon inhalation and contracts upon exhalation. As Jiang Weiqiao 蔣維橋, or Master Yinshi, an early forerunner of the Qigong movement, already observes in his *Yinshizi jingzuo fa* 因是子靜坐法 (Quiet Sitting with Master Yinshi), published in 1914:

> In ordinary people, the respiration never expands or con-
> tracts the lungs to their full capacity. They only use the up-
> per section of the lungs while their lower section hardly ever
> is employed at all. Because of this they cannot gain the full
> advantage of deep breathing, their blood and body fluids are
> not refreshed, and the various diseases gain easy entry. (Lu
> 1964, 171; Kohn 1993, 86)

Breathing only as far as the chest causes the entire breathing process
to speed up. Instead of ten or twelve deep and relaxed breaths per
minute, people take sixteen or more. The heart accordingly beats
faster; it begins to work overtime and comes to wear out sooner.
Heart disease and cardio-pulmonary conditions are the eventual result. Besides, this shallow breathing prevents sufficient amounts of
oxygen for reaching the body's cells. Instead of exchanging fresh oxygen for old carbon dioxide in the lungs and thereby giving new energy
to the body, people only release a little and maintain an unhealthy
amount of gaseous toxins within—what the ancients call "stale *qi*"
and link with the ingestion of the five flavors.

Today, medical science says that this causes the blood to become more
acidic and tension to build up, which in turn stimulates the hypo-
thalamus and pituitary glands and leads to the release of stress hor-
mones such as cortisole and adrenaline. They in their turn fuel the
sense of urgency, tension, and anxiety, which creates a yet shallower
and more rapid form of breathing—a vicious circle that leads to disease and death (see Loehr and Migdow 1986; Farhi 1996).

Learning how to breathe deeply, consciously, and in a relaxed environment has immediate and direct health benefits. The six healing
breaths, when seen in this light, are a highly efficient way of increasing people's awareness of their bodies, reducing stress levels, and developing a healthier life. Whether undertaken as simple exercises
purely for medical reasons or for more spiritual purposes in conjunction with meditations and healing exercises, they provide an easy and
efficient way toward balance and harmony. The different models developed over the centuries, the various symptoms associated with the
organs, and the many different methods accompanying the practice
all bear witness to the basic efficacy and importance of breathing
practice—from the depths of Chinese antiquity to the forefront of
twenty-first century body cultivation.

Bibliography

Barrett, T. H. 1982. "Daoist and Buddhist Mysteries in the Interpretation of the *Tao-te-ching*," *Journal of the Royal Asiatic Society* 1 (1982), 35-43.

Bokenkamp, Stephen. 1997. *Early Daoist Scriptures*. With a contribution by Peter Nickerson. Berkeley: University of California Press.

Campany, Robert F. 2002. *To Live As Long As Heaven and Earth: A Translation and Study of Ge Hong's Traditions of Divine Transcendents*. Berkeley: University of California Press.

Chan, Alan. 1991. *Two Visions of the Way: A Study of the Wang Pi and the Ho-shang-kung Commentaries on the Laozi*. Albany: State University of New York Press.

Chia, Mantak, and Maneewan Chia. 1993. *Awaken Healing Light of the Tao*. Huntington, NY: Healing Tao Books.

DeBruyn, Pierre-Henry. 2000. "Daoism in the Ming (1368-1644)." In *Daoism Handbook*, edited by Livia Kohn, 594-622. Leiden: E. Brill.

Despeux, Catherine. 1988. *La moélle du phénix rouge: Santé et longue vie dans la Chine du seiziéme siècle*. Paris: Editions Trédaniel.

_____. 1989. "Gymnastics: The Ancient Tradition." In *Taoist Meditation and Longevity Techniques*, edited by Livia Kohn, 223-61. Ann Arbor: University of Michigan, Center for Chinese Studies Publications.

_____. 1995. "L'expiration des six souffles d'après les sources du Canon taoïque: un procédé classique du Qigong." In *Hommage a Kwong Hing Foon: Etudes d'histoire culturelle de la Chine*, edited by Jean-Pierre Diény,129-63. Paris: Collège du France, Institut des Hautes Etudes Chinoises.

_____, and Frederic Obringer, eds. 1997. *La maladie dans la Chine médiévale: La toux*. Paris: Editions L'Harmattan.

DeWoskin, Kenneth J. 1983. *Doctors, Diviners, and Magicians of Ancient China*. New York: Columbia University Press.

Ding Guangdi 丁光迪. 1993. *Zhubing yuanhou lun yangsheng fang daoyin fa yanjiu* 諸病源候論養生方導引法研究. Beijing: Renmin weisheng.

Engelhardt, Ute. 1996. "Zur Bedeutung der Atmung im Qigong." *Chinesische Medizin* 1/1996: 17-23.

_____. 2001. "*Daoyin tu* und *Yinshu*: Neue Erkenntnisse über die Übungen zur Lebenspflege in der frühen Han-Zeit." *Monumenta Serica* 49: 213-26.

Farhi, Donna. 1996. *The Breathing Book*. New York: Henry Holt.

Graham, A. C. 1986. *Chuang-tzu: The Inner Chapters*. London: Allan & Unwin.

Harper, Donald. 1998. *Early Chinese Medical Manuscripts: The Mawangdui Medical Manuscripts*. London: Wellcome Asian Medical Monographs.

Homann, Rolf. 1971. *Die wichtigsten Körpergottheiten im Huang-t'ing-ching*. Göppingen: Alfred Kümmerle.

Hoshino Minoru 星野稔.1985. *Kikō kenkōhō* 氣功健康法. Tokyo: Nihon bungeisha, 1985.

Huang, Jane, and Michael Wurmbrand. 1987. *The Primordial Breath: Ancient Chinese Ways of Prolonging Life Through Breath*. Torrance, Cal.: Original Books.

Kaltenmark, Maxime. 1953. *Le Lie-sien tchouan*. Peking: Universite de Paris Publications.

Kim, Tawn. 1979. *Les exercices secrets des moines taoïstes*. Paris: Guy Trédaniel.

Kohn, Livia 1993. "Quiet Sitting with Master Yinshi: Medicine and Religion in Modern China." *Zen Buddhism Today* 10: 79-95. Reprint in *Living with the Dao* (www.threepinespress.com).

_____. 1998. *God of the Dao: Lord Lao in History and Myth*. University of Michigan, Center for Chinese Studies.

_____. forthcoming. *Chinese Healing Exercises*. Magdalena, NM: Three Pines Press.

Kroll, Paul W. 1996. "Body Gods and Inner Vision: *The Scripture of the Yellow Court*. In *Religions of China in Practice*, edited by Donald S. Lopez Jr., 149-55. Princeton: Princeton University Press.

Leong, Patricia. "The *Daoyin tu*." Paper presented at the conference on "Daoist Cultivation Traditional Models and Contemporary Practices," Camp Sealth, Vashon Island, 2001.

Loehr, James E., and Jeffrey A. Migdow. 1986. *Breathe In, Breathe Out: Inhale Energy and Exhale Stress by Guiding and Controlling Your Breathing.* Alexandria, VA: Time Life Books.

Loon, Piet van der. 1984. *Taoist Books in the Libraries of the Sung Period.* London: Oxford Oriental Institute.

Lu, Kuan-yü. 1964. *The Secrets of Chinese Meditation.* London: Rider.

Ma Chun 馬春. 1983. *Majia qigong* 馬家氣功. Shanxi: Renmin chubanshe.

Ma Jixing 馬繼興. 1992. *Mawangdui guyishu kaoshi* 馬王堆古醫書考釋. Changsha: Renmin.

Maspero, Henri. 1981. *Taoism and Chinese Religion.* Translated by Frank Kierman. Amherst: University of Massachusetts Press.

Miura, Kunio. 1989. "The Revival of *Qi:* Qigong in Contemporary China." In *Taoist Meditation and Longevity Techniques*, edited by L. Kohn, 329-58. Ann Arbor: University of Michigan, Center for Chinese Studies Publications.

Miyazawa Masayori 宮澤正順. 1984. "Dōsho no ikkōsatsu" 道樞の一考察. *Tōhō shūkyō* 東方宗教 63: 22-35.

Mugitani Kunio 麥谷邦夫. 1987. "Yōsei enmei roku kunchu" 養性延命錄訓注. *Report of the Study Group on Traditional Chinese Longevity Techniques*, no. 3. Tokyo: Mombushō.

Needham, Joseph, et al. 1983. *Science and Civilisation in China*, vol. V.5: Spagyrical Discovery and Invention—Physiological Alchemy. Cambridge: Cambridge University Press.

Rao Zongyi 饒宗頤. 1992. *Laozi xianger zhu jiaojian* 老子想爾注校箋. Shanghai: Wenyi.

Ren Jiyu 任繼愈 and Zhong Zhaopeng 鐘肇鵬, eds. 1991. *Daozang tiyao* 道藏提要. Beijing: Zhongguo shehui kexue chubanshe.

Robinet, Isabelle. 1989. "Visualization and Ecstatic Flight in Shangqing Taoism." In *Taoist Meditation and Longevity Techniques*, edited by Livia Kohn, 157-90. Ann Arbor: University of Michigan, Center for Chinese Studies Publications.

_____. 1993. *Taoist Meditation.* Translated by Norman Girardot and Julian Pas. Albany: State University of New York Press.

Sakade Yoshinobu 扳出祥伸. 1986a. "Chō Tan 'Yōsei yōshu' itsubun to sono shisō" 張湛養生要集跡文とその思想. *Tōhōshukyō* 東方宗教 68: 1-24.

_____. 1986b. "The Daoist Character of the 'Chapter on Nourishing Life' of the *Ishimpō*." *Kansai daigaku bunka ronshū* 關西大學文化論集 1986: 775-798.

_____. 1986c. "Kaisetsu: dōin no enkaku" 解說：導引の沿革. In *Dōin taiyō* 導引提要, edited by Kitamura Yoshikatsu 喜田村利且, 1-41. Tokyo: Taniguchi shoten.

Sawada Mizuhō 澤田瑞惠. 1974. "Kō no genryu" 嘯の源流. *Tōhōshūkyō* 東方宗教 44:1-14.

Schipper, Kristofer M. 1975. *Concordance du Houang-t'ing king*. Paris: Publications de l'Ecole Française d'Extrême-Orient.

_____. 1980. *Concordance du Yun ki ki kian*. 2 vols. Paris: Publications de l'Ecole Française d'Extrême-Orient.

Stein, Stephan. 1999. *Zwischen Heil und Heilung: Zur frühen Tradition des Yangsheng in China*. Uelzen: Medizinisch-Literarische Verlagsgesellschaft.

Sun Simiao 孫思邈. 1983. *Qianjin yifang* 千金翼方. Beijing: Renmin weisheng.

_____. 1992. *Qianjin yaofang* 千金要方. Beijing: Renmin weisheng.

Switkin, Walter. 1987. *Immortality: A Taoist Text of Macrobiotics*. San Francisco: H. S. Dakin Company.

Tsuchiya, Masaaki. 2002. "Confession of Sins and Awareness of Self in the *Taiping jing*." In *Daoist Identity: History, Lineage, and Ritual*, edited by Livia Kohn and Harold D. Roth, 39-57. Honolulu: University of Hawaii Press.

Unschuld, Paul U. 1985. *Medicine in China: A History of Ideas*. Berkeley: University of California Press.

Wenwu 文物. 1990. "Zhangjiashan Hanjian *Yinshu* shiwen" 張家山漢簡引書釋文. *Wenwu* 文物 10/1990: 82-86.

Chapter Three

Ingestion, Digestion, and Regestation:

The Complexities of *Qi*-Absorption

STEPHEN JACKOWICZ

Daoist cultivation practices include a battery of techniques based on the manipulation of *qi* for the purpose of spiritual change. One category of these techniques is termed *fuqi* 服氣 or "absorption of *qi*." In modern Chinese medicine, *fuqi* is used without an intrinsically spiritual component, however, as Ute Engelhardt observes, "during the early beginnings of what we would call Chinese medicine, perhaps even before the development of acupuncture, these techniques of nourishing life must have been of equal importance as moxibustion and drug therapy" (1989, 272). Let us therefore examine the manipulation of *qi* in the medical as well as Daoist spiritual contexts to better understand the rich complexity of theory behind Daoist cultivation.

Eating Qi

Historically, there are many ways to manipulate *qi* in relation to the body. Among the multiplicity of subtle variations of this *qi* manipulation, I will first look at a practice known as *shiqi* 食氣 or "eating *qi*." Doing so, I provide a backdrop for the examination of *fuqi* as well as a contrast to the modern understanding.

The term *shiqi* first appears in a collection of texts known as the Mawangdui 馬王堆 manuscripts found in 1973 in a tomb in Changsha, Hunan, that was closed in 168 B.C.E. The tomb contained a large assortment of texts, many of which deal with medicine and self-cultivation. Among them is the *Quegu shiqi* 卻穀食氣 (Abstaining from Grains and Eating *Qi*; see Harper 1998). It deals mainly with techniques of eliminating grains and ordinary foodstuffs from the diet and replacing them with medicinal herbs and *qi* through special breathing exercises. The text repeatedly contrasts "those who eat *qi*" with "those who eat grain" and explains this in cosmological terms. It says: "Those who eat grain eat what is square; those who eat *qi* eat what is round. Round is Heaven; square is Earth" (Harper 1998, 130).

Shiqi in this text thus literally means to "eat *qi*," that is to ingest *qi* instead of eating food. Donald Harper in his translation of the manuscripts observes that this interpretation of the term is unique to the *Quegu shiqi* and notes that "the contrast is not made elsewhere in the Mawangdui and Zhangjiashan macrobiotic hygiene texts; 'eating vapor' is simply the term for breath cultivation and the regular consumption of drink and food is assumed" (1998, 130).

That is to say, in the Han dynasty (206 B.C.E.-220 C.E.), immortality practices developed that made the method of grain elimination in conjunction with attempts to eat pure *qi* more general. There is evidence of individuals attempting to alter their physiological state and achieve a state of spiritual transcendence making them into other-worldly beings known as *xian* 仙, immortals or transcendents. These people strove to extend physical life and attain mysterious and magical powers. Beyond that, they hoped to reach a type of spiritual coherence after death that allowed them to maintain a personal consciousness, to live in pure spirit existence, and—if desired—to intercede in mortal affairs while standing outside the flow of time. The practices associated with immortality are documented from the Han dynasty onward; later they became increasingly ornate and formed the basis for much of the Daoist religion (see Kohn 1989).

The *Quegu shiqi* focuses on three aspects of the immortal endeavor. It prescribes the substitution of tongue-fern (*pyrossia*) for normal foodstuffs, an herb that is used today to promote urination but was historically used while fasting to maintain normal urinary output and avoid toxidosis from the restricted intake (Bensky 1986, 140). It also suggests the use of breathing practices for *qi*-regulation as the body adjusts to the transformation, especially of the *xu* 呴 and *chui* 吹 breaths. An early reference to focused breathing for *qi*-manipulation, the text already notes that *xu* cools the liver while *chui* warms the kidneys.

In Chinese medical terms, the liver is associated with the phase wood which governs the phase earth in the controlling cycle. When restricting the diet, the earth organs of the body will be free of their normal duties. Due to this, the spleen-yang will not be required to digest the grain qi, which means that the relative amount of upward driving qi in the body is increased. The nature of liver-wood is to ascend and thus there will be an overabundance of upward flowing qi. This manifests in the body as heat. The xu sound aids the liver in its function of ensuring the free qi-flow in the body, allowing the heat to vent. Another way to counterbalance the heat is to strengthen the kidneys, the seat of qi of the phase water. The kidneys are also the body's base of power and the reservoir of the will. Fasting requires just these qualities, making the practice of exhaling with chui a necessity. Aside from the emphasis on these two breaths, a third focus of the text is on eating qi at certain times of the year to take in a specific type. In this context, it outlines how qi becomes a substitute for food and is ingested just like food.

Eating qi can, therefore, be understood as both a general way of referring to breathing practices and the specific method of substituting qi for food, especially if undertaken at certain times of day and year that allow access to the different types of qi. Taking these ideas together, we can see that the use of the verb shi, "to eat," carries a fairly mechanical component with it. The substance eaten is qi rather than the grosser foodstuffs which cause the body's decay, but the technical process is the same. In effect, there is no transformation of the inner mechanics of the body. The lungs continue to breathe and the stomach still digests. But the ability of the organs is perfected to a higher level of efficiency, allowing the avoidance of coarse foodstuffs.

To understand this process better, let us look at Chinese medicine. According to this, there exists a fundamental distinction in the physiology before birth and after birth. Before birth, the body is considered to be nourished by prenatal and primordial qi, derived from parental and universal qi which directly infuse the embryo. This type of metabolism does not engage the digestive tract. Rather, nutrients enter through the umbilicus, which to the traditional mindset is related to the lower elixir field, an energy center in the abdomen named after the alchemical crucible in which the elixir of life was concocted. Once people are born, however, that direct connection to the universal flow is restricted and they enter a phase where they are nourished by postnatal qi. Postnatal qi is derived from food, air, and water.

The postnatal metabolism utilizes the lungs and spleen and their associated meridians to convert worldly materials into useable *qi*. The lungs receive breath from the nose. While drawn in through the nose, this is called *qingqi* 清氣 or "pure *qi*," but once it reaches the lungs it is known as *kongqi* 空氣, "empty *qi*." From the lungs, it descends to the kidneys. At the same time, the stomach grinds up any food after it has been ingested through the mouth, preparing it for the spleen to extract its *qi*. Known as *guqi* 穀氣 or "grain *qi*," this ascends to the middle elixir field in the chest where the fire of the heart, driven by the essence of the kidneys (which is enhanced by empty *qi*), helps the Upper Heater to transform it into *zongqi* 宗氣 or "ancestral *qi*."

Ancestral *qi* next combines with the primordial *qi* already stored in the depth of the person to form *zhenqi* 真氣 or "true *qi*." This in turn divides and moves on to return again, in its new form, to the lungs and the spleen. In the lungs, true *qi* is divided into meridian *qi* (*maiqi* 脈氣), i.e., the *qi* in the meridians of the body, and defensive *qi* (*weiqi* 衛氣) which circulates close to the body's surface. In the spleen, it becomes nutritive *qi* (*yingqi* 營氣) which flows in the deeper interstices.

In the cosmology of ancient China, both pure *qi* and empty *qi* are an emanation of the energy of Heaven, that is, yang in nature. Empty *qi* follows the laws of yang and moves downward, issuing from Heaven and sinking toward Earth. A downward moving form of yang energy, empty *qi* assists the lungs' function of descending *qi* in the body. Similarly, grain *qi* as won from food is an emanation of Earth. It has the same nature as Earth-yin, namely to flow upward. As grain *qi* naturally moves up, it matches the functional tendency of spleen-yang, which raises it to the Upper Heater.

Now, as and when empty *qi* and grain *qi* come together at the heart, the beating of the heart, a direct expression of heart-fire, serves as a transformative force to synthesize them into ancestral *qi*. This transformation corresponds to the formation of a societal unit in the human world. A yang force (male, superior, older) melds with a yin force (female, inferior, younger). They are wedded together by the agglutinative fire of the heart (love, caring, compassion), and a family or other social unit is formed. This social part of the vision is echoed in the term ancestral *qi*, reflecting that our parents are our ancestors. However, this ancestral *qi* cannot be used directly by the body. Rather, it has to merge with primordial *qi*, the source *qi* of the body. Only when the *qi* has reached this conjunction is it transformed by the fire of the heart into true *qi*—the *qi* that is truly human and can finally be used by the body.

Another layer of the terminological distinctions implicit in this second transformation is that the basic energies of empty *qi* and grain *qi* follow the laws of yin and yang in the universe, yin going up and yang going down. However, the *qi* in the human body follows a different configuration. Here yin sinks down and yang floats up. The union of empty *qi* and grain *qi* alone does not imbue either of them with the necessary human *qi*-orientation. Rather, their transformation in the form of ancestral *qi* must be combined with the original, primordial *qi* in the body and only then acquires the "rotated" or "reversed" nature it needs to function within. The combined synthesis of the various forms of *qi* in the human body thus allows the downward driving yang of nature to be reverted back to Heaven and the upward driving yin of nature to be rotated back to Earth (see Fig. 1).

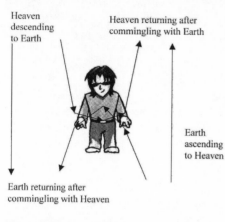

Heaven descending to Earth

Heaven returning after commingling with Earth

Earth ascending to Heaven

Earth returning after commingling with Heaven

Fig. 1: Heaven and Earth in the human being

This shows just how the purpose of normal human physiology lies in its role as a pivotal meeting ground of Heaven and Earth. Here the two poles of existence co-mingle and acknowledge each other, then are directed back from where they came, each having partaken of and intimately learned the other. Intrinsic within the mundane physiology of the unascended human being, therefore, is the fundamental spirituality of existence, an intimate state of interwovenness between the ascended and the unascended.

Daoist spiritual practices, when seen from this perspective, seek to redefine the nature of the intimacy between human physiology and universal Dao. Immortality or transcendence accordingly is a matter of retooling the mechanics of the body and thereby the spirit. Reality is not rejected per se, but the ability to reorganize the physiologic relationship of the human to the universe implies that the rules of mundane existence are only apparently fixed. Daoist spirituality ventures to change the nature of the absorption of *qi* in the body, thereby transforming the individual's role in the whole of creation.

Eating *qi* does not go this far. It is a more basic practice which can be described as a simple substitution. The mechanics of physiology, breathing and digestion, remain the same but one switches to a cleaner burning type of fuel, to a more refined and purer energetic connection to the Dao. The engine is unchanged but the output increases due to the efficiency. This changes in the practice of *qi* absorption.

Absorbing Qi

The practice of absorbing *qi* first appears in Daoist and medical literature in the Tang dynasty when immortality and long life practices were integrated into a coherent system. The techniques and concepts reflect the prevalent medical knowledge of the time and focus on maintaining health, avoiding disease, and extending life.

A key document that describes the practice is the *Yangxing yanming lu* 養性延命錄 (On Nourishing Inner Nature and Extending Life, DZ 838), ascribed to the physician and Daoist master Sun Simiao 孫思邈 (610-693). It describes longevity practices under six headings:

1. General Guidelines, including ethical principles;
2. Dietary Practices, e.g., the avoidance of spoilt or preserved foods;
3. Behavioral Moderation, such as getting enough sleep;
4. Absorption of *Qi*, i.e., breathing practices and inner visualizations;
5. Healing Exercises and Self-massages, ways to stimulate energy flow in the body;
6. Sexual Practices, enhancing *qi* through intimate contact and sexual refinement.[1]

As the preface points out, the text combines materials from various earlier sources to provide a collection of resources on extending life:

> Let your mind wander freely in emptiness and tranquility, rest all thinking, remain in nonaction, absorb *qi* after the *zi* hour [midnight], practice exercises in a secluded chamber, collect and nurture the self without defilement, restrict your diet and take herbal medicines: by doing all this you can reach a long life of a hundred years. (1a)

---

[1] Sections 2 and 3 are translated in Switkin 1987; Section 4 is presented in Jackowicz 2003. The entire text exists in an annotated Japanese translation (Mugitani 1987).

The text works dominantly with inner nature, which allows practitioners to become immortal if they cultivate it properly. It also focuses on the preservation and extension of life, so that they have the time to reach immortality.

Another classic on the subject is the *Fuqi jingyi lun* 服氣精義論 (The Essential Meaning of the Absorption of *Qi*, DZ 277, 830) by Sima Chengzhen 司馬承禎 (647-735), famous patriarch of Highest Clarity.[2] This work divides longevity practices into nine forms:

1. The Five Sprouts, i.e., meditative absorption of the *qi* of the five directions;
2. Absorption of *Qi*, breathing practices and internal *qi* circulation;
3. Healing Exercises, body movements and stretches;
4. Talisman Water, the drinking of talisman ashes dissolved in water;
5. Medicines, the replacement of ordinary food with herbs and minerals;
6. Practical Precautions, the observation of behavioral and religious taboos;
7. The Five Organs, visualizing the body gods and calming the inner organs;
8. Healing Diseases, taking control over the different forms of *qi* to secure health;
9. Diagnostics, learning to understand the symptoms of disharmony and the patterns of the body.

The focus is both medical and spiritual in that the text emphasizes the complete curing of all ailments and conditions, but also presents ways to stop eating and completely transform the body's metabolism toward immortality. The preface outlines the theory behind it:

> *Qi* is the origin of the embryo and the root of the body. As soon as the embryo has taken birth, the primordial essence begins to disperse; as soon as the body begins to move, its fundamental substance gradually decays. For this reason, we take in *qi* to stabilize essence and preserve *qi* to refine the body. If essence is in fullness, spirit is complete; if the body is stable, destiny is extended. If both origin and root are firm, you can live forever. (1a; Engelhardt 1987, 99)

---

[2] An earlier edition is contained in the Daoist encyclopedia *Yunji qiqian* 雲笈七籤 (Seven Tablets from a Cloudy Satchel, DZ 1032) which dates from the eleventh century (ch. 57). The text is available in a German translation (Engelhardt 1987). For further discussion, see Engelhardt 1989.

This makes it clear that *qi* is the key force in the body that creates and enriches life, and that by cultivating and renewing *qi* one can stabilize the other forces and eventually reach the perfection of spirit and attain long life and immortality.

Both the *Fuqi jingyi lun* and the *Yangxing yanming lu* agree that *qi* is the fundamental cosmic energy in the body that manifests in a number of different forces: spirit (*shen* 神), essence (*jing* 精), and the heart-mind (*xin* 心). The interplay between these forces gives rise to different states of health, emotions, and mentation. Through their proper manipulation, moreover, one can not only perfect health and attain long life, but also can transcend the physical limitations of the body and become an immortal. However, this is no simple task. The aspirant may take herbal medicines, practice controlled breathing, perform healing exercises, and sit in absorptive meditation to promote the proper flow of cosmic *qi*. This takes time, so one has to first pursue the goal of living a long life before one can seek transformation into an otherworldly being. By living for the requisite time and practicing the proper methods, one eventually reaches immortality.

Both texts also agree that part of the absorption of *qi* is, as in eating *qi*, to become free of ordinary foodstuffs and to gain the ability to live on pure *qi*. They both outline concrete methods for doing so; beginning by emphasizing that one should first cure all diseases and unhealthy conditions. The *Fuqi jingyi lun* says:

> If you want to absorb *qi*, first heal all bodily ailments and illnesses to allow the organs and viscera to open up in free flow and the limbs to be at rest and in harmony. Even if there are no specific old ailments, take certain medicinal supplements.

> If your body is sensitive to cold and heat, for example, use an anti-phlegm concoction. To open and empty the stomach and intestines, a laxative is beneficial. To remove obstructions and hindrances [in the *qi*-flow], use an expectorants as discussed below [in the section on drugs].

> Once your breathing is completely even, stop all supplements, then undergo a hundred-day fast. All this helps to purify the body and disciplines the will. In the meantime, gradually lessen the amount of food you take, increasingly staying away from all sour and salty substances. Continue to take moisturizing items, though, including drugs like poria fungus; steamed, dried sesame; and the like. All this is very good to prepare for abstaining from grains. (5b-6a)

Similarly, the *Yangxing yanming lu* stresses that one should take good care to eliminate obstructions and harmful patterns. However, rather than recommending the taking of herbal remedies, it notes that one can effect cures with the help of the circulation of *qi.* It says:

> Circulate the *qi* in order to expel the hundred ailments. Follow it wherever it is needed and develop clear awareness there. If your head hurts, become aware of your head; if your foot hurts, become aware of your foot, using harmonized *qi* to attack the pain. From one moment to the next, it will dissolve by itself.
>
> If the *qi* is internally cold or frozen, enclose it [by holding the breath] to cause sweating. When sweat emerges it regulates the body, and the cold will be dissolved. Circulating and enclosing the *qi* are the essentials of healing the body. . . . Circulating the *qi* makes people develop superior *qi.* Anyone wishing to learn this method should always use a step-by-step approach. (2.1b-2a)

The text also recommends that one eat a small amount, because over-indulgence will lead the *qi* to rebel and cause improper circulation. This admonition echoes the *Huangdi neijing suwen* 黃帝內經素問 (The Yellow Emperor's Inner Classic, Simple Questions; see Eckmann 1996; Ni 1995; Wu and Wu 1999), which describes the spleen being taxed by over-consumption and the necessity to balance the five flavors. By keeping amounts low, the body's *qi* is able to circulate. Another good thing to do for the circulation of *qi* is the practice of simple body movements in coordination with the breath, known as *daoyin*, literally "guiding [the *qi*] and stretching [the body]," which continue in modern Qigong.

The mind in all these practices should be calm and concentrated, with intention directed toward health and immortality (2.1a). The mind is the seat of consciousness, which traditionally resides in the heart. The intention is the 'autopilot' that allows the body to maintain a number of activities at the same time—traditionally associated with the spleen. This implies that a unity of mind and body takes place in such a way that the dissociation of the psyche and anatomy, a regular part of daily consciousness in most people, would end. This means that the mind leads the intention to keep the body healthy, obviating the need for medicine. It also leads to the use of the mind in active visualization of *qi* as it circulates through the body.

Another aspect of healing as a preliminary practice for the absorption of *qi* is the avoidance of what the *Yangxing yanming lu* calls the five labors which will give rise to stress in six different areas of the body. The text says:

> The five labors are [creating exertion through] will, thinking, mind, worry, and fatigue. These five labors create six forms of extreme pressure in the body, to wit, in *qi*, blood, tendons, bones, essence, and bone marrow. These six forms of extreme pressure in turn cause the seven injuries which transform into the seven pains. The seven pains create disease. (2.3b)

The text does not spell out what the seven pains are, but it describes the process of disease origination as an increase in *xieqi* ("wayward *qi*"), which will primarily affect the two key organs of the heart and kidneys. *Xieqi* 邪氣 is the opposite of *zhengqi* 正氣 ("proper *qi*"), a division of *qi* that forms a key concept for the correct understanding of the absorption of *qi*.

What, then, do these two terms refer to? Most generally, they indicate the way *qi* flows in the body—any kind of *qi*, empty, grain, ancestral, or true *qi*. *Zhengqi* or "proper *qi*" indicates the presence of a strong vital energy in a smooth, harmonious, and active flow. This is ideal, a state when *qi* flows freely, thereby creating harmony in the body and a balanced state of being. This personal health is further matched by health in nature, defined as regular weather patterns and the absence of disasters. It is also present as health in society in the peaceful coexistence among families, clans, villages, and states.

Since the term *zheng* is not limited to the medical context but also indicates the correct rhythm of nature, the proper way of living in society, the orthodox attitude of conforming with the government, and the upright position of a proper citizen and family member, it has been rendered in a number of different ways even when used medically. Some translators, wishing to maintain the moral and social context, have chosen a socially inspired rendition, such as "upright *qi*" (see Unschuld 1985; Wiseman and Boss 1990), while others prefer a more medical, technical word, such as "orthopathic" (Porkert 1974; Sivin 1988; Needham et al. 2000).

The opposite of *zhengqi* is *xieqi* or "wayward *qi*," similarly rendered differently. It can be called "deviant *qi*," "secessionist *qi*," or "evil *qi*," integrating its larger social and ethical application, or be translated as "heteropathic *qi*" or "pathogenic *qi*," using Latin-based technical and medical terms. Whatever its appellation, *xieqi* is *qi* that has lost the harmonious pattern of flow and no longer supports the dynamic forces of change. Whereas *zhengqi* moves in a steady, harmonious rhythm and effects daily renewal, helping health and long life, *xieqi*, is disorderly and dysfunctional, and creates change that violates the normal order. *Xieqi* appears when *qi* begins to move either too fast or too slow, is excessive or depleted, or creates rushes or obstructions. It disturbs the regular flow and causes ailments. According to the *Yangxing yanming lu*, people affected by *xieqi* have the following symptoms:

> They are confused and likely to forget things, always griev-
> ous and injured, do not enjoy their food and drink, and do
> not gain weight and robustness. Their facial complexion is
> without glossiness, their hair turns white and they wither
> away. When this becomes serious, they are easily injured by
> great wind. They will be stooped and brittle, their tendons
> restricting the four limbs from agility and pulling together
> the hundred joints. There will be blockages of the dia-
> phragm, numbness in the body, shortness of breath, and
> many aches in the waist and back. (2.3b)

It is quite impossible for people to be completely free from *xieqi* as they live in the ordinary world, and the body typically consists of a combination of both correct and wayward flowing *qi* (see Fig. 2). Commonly the *qi* is in good order in the womb before birth, nourished by the universe directly through prenatal *qi* which effuses the kidneys. However, after birth the imperfect nature of food, air, and water in combination with attendant trauma, as well as disease-causing agents of the phe-nomenal world, make *xieqi* an active part of life. Dysfunctional and impure, people can no longer access the universal *qi* which nourished them in the womb. Relying on the spleen and lungs as the main avenue to replenish energy via postnatal *qi*, they will surely die and rot as their putrid fecal waste shows.

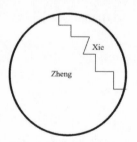

Fig. 2: Forms of *qi* flow

This is where the absorption of *qi* comes in. Not only a way to replace ordinary nourishment with *qi*, it is a method to completely internalize *qi* circulation. It works by shutting down the lungs and spleen, thereby forcing the body to return to its original pattern of the kidney system as the primary source of nourishment. The kidneys, awakened from their dormancy, are forced to reconnect with the primordial *qi* of the universe, and the internal mechanism of the body is transformed (see Figs. 3a and 3b).

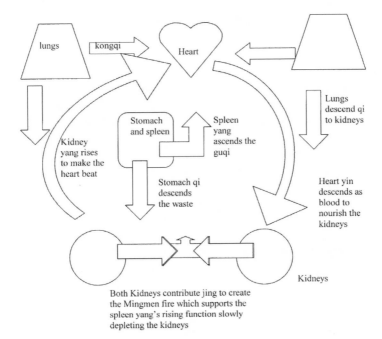

Fig. 3a. Postnatal Metabolism

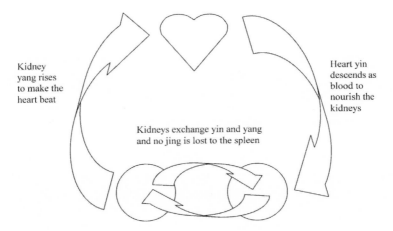

Fig. 3b. Metabolism after self-cultivation

The Practice

The absorption of *qi* is a complex method that consists of several phases to be undertaken after the body has been cured of all major ailments and is already used to taking herbal medicines and *qi* rather than solid food. As the *Fuqi jingyi lun* points out, it should be performed in a quiet, secluded room that has windows in all directions and is both comfortably warm and well ventilated. The best time to commence the practice is in the beginning of the lunar month, after the third and before the eighth day. Practitioners enter the chamber around midnight, when the period of rising or living *qi* (*shengqi* 生氣) begins, loosen their hair and clothing, burn incense, face east, and sit or kneel in quiet meditation to calm their thoughts and concentrate on the matter at hand. They then open the *qi* flow through the joints by performing a simple exercise sequence.

These preliminaries accomplished, they lie down flat on their backs. As the *Fuqi jingyi lun* says:

> The mattress should be thick and warm. Cover yourself according to the prevailing temperature so that you are comfortable. It is best if especially the lower body, from hips to feet, is nicely warm on both the right and the left sides. If you want your neck support low, make it lower than the back. If you want it high, set it to be in line with the body so that trunk, head, and neck are on the same level. (6b)

In this position, practitioners begin by breathing slowly and consciously, inhaling through the nose and exhaling through the mouth. They then practice swallowing the *qi*. This involves taking in long, deep inhalations through the nose and allowing the breath to reach the mouth, where it mingles with the saliva. This mixture is then consciously swallowed through the gullet and into the lungs, where it is held for a little while. To conclude, practitioners exhale softly through the mouth with lips slightly open. As the *Yangxing yanming lu* says, citing the *Yuanyang jing* 元陽經 (Scripture of Primordial Yang):

> Always take in the *qi* through the nose, hold it in the mouth, and rinse with it until it is full. Allow it to envelope the tongue, lips, and teeth, then swallow it. If you can do one thousand swallowings like this in one day and night, this is most excellent. (2.1a)

An alternative way of practice is by inhaling three, five, or seven breaths consecutively, then mixing and swallowing these while exhaling only briefly (Maspero 1981, 474). The goal is to enrich the breath with saliva as another form of *qi* and to enter this potent mixture into the lungs. With time practitioners will, as the *Fuqi jingyi lun* says, "feel the lungs expanding and enlarging, and thus know that the right measure has been reached" (7a). The text also admonishes to practice this with due moderation, making sure that inhalation and exhalation are even and harmonious at all times.

Swallowing *qi* is not unlike eating *qi* in that clean outside air is entered consciously into the body and swallowed in conjunction with saliva. It is meant to reach mainly the lungs, but it will obviously also flow into the stomach and spleen area, where it can substitute for ordinary nourishment. From here, however, practitioners move on to the next part of *qi*-absorption, which is quite different. It is called "enclosing the *qi*" (*biqi* 閉氣). The *Yangxing yanming lu* describes it as follows:

> Lie down flat on your back, close your eyes, and curl your hands into fists.
>> Note: Curling your hands into fists is making fists like an infant would, with the four fingers enclosing the thumb.
> Enclose the *qi* and do not breathe. Mentally count to 200, then expel the *qi* by exhaling through the mouth.
>
> As you breathe like this for an increasing number of days, you will find your body, spirit, and all the five organs being at peace. If you can enclose the *qi* to the count of 250, your Flowery Canopy will be bright.
>> Note: The Flowery Canopy is the eyebrows.
> Your eyes and ears will be perceptive and clear, and your body will be light and free from disease; nothing wayward [*xie*] will bother you any more. (2b)

In other words, the practice involves holding the breath in for an extended period—a count of 200 or more comes to three or four minutes—while also tightly closing the various other *qi*-openings of the body, such as the eyes and mouth, the palms of the hands and the soles of the feet. Presumably the perineum at the anus is also pulled in, preventing *qi* from leaving the body through any major orifice. More specifically, by encasing the thumb in the palm the five organs are reorganized.

According to the traditional Daoist attribution of the fingers to the organs, the pinkie relates to the kidneys, the ring finger to the liver, the middle finger to the heart, and the index finger to the lungs. The thumb, which is enclosed, corresponds to the spleen, the moving force of digestion and the seat of the generation of postnatal *qi*. This system of correspondence is also activated in the creation of sacred hand signs or *mudras*, which prescribe how the fingers should be held in intricate patterns that reflect the internal changes in the practitioner's body while also serving as a tool to effect these changes (see Mitamura 2002). The tradition holds that high levels of spiritual attainment lead to the spontaneous performance of these hand signs or finger knittings and that, vice versa, it is beneficial for the attainment of higher level to mimic the hand positions (see Zhang 1996).

In the absorption of *qi*, practitioners enclose the thumb within the other fingers to effect a sympathetic magical response, that is, to transform a microcosmic environment which has been charged through its connection to the macrocosm by either natural correspondence or by invoking of the practitioner's will and concentration. Doing so, adepts shut down the digestive tract and thereby divorce themselves from the nourishment of postnatal *qi*. Curling the hands into fists and closing the eyes, practitioners hold the breath and thereby shut off the lungs, again disconnecting from the postnatal sources of *qi*, forcing the body to revert to prenatal forms of *qi* circulation.

The first sign of success is the body being permeated with sweat. Sweat is traditionally linked with the heart and the kidneys. Its ap-

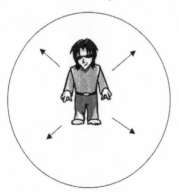

pearance indicates that the kidneys, associated with the phase of water, have succeeded in effusing to the heart, the phase of fire, thereby producing the equivalent of steam (see Zhang 1996). This primordial vapor emanates from the center of the body and normalizes the internal reactions, converting the *xieqi* of the organs into *zhengqi*, or driving out the *xieqi* which had invaded from the outside by allowing it to be.

Fig. 4. Expelling *xie* components

The individual returns to the primordial state of being and is like the embryo, but instead of being supported by a mother's body, he or she is now nourished in the womb of the universe, the body corrected to be only *zhengqi* (see Fig. 4). The universe is *zheng* and the individual partakes of its nature, so that even what was formerly considered *xie* is now part of universal correctness. The practitioner in his or her body has returned to the stage of the primordial egg, from which the comic giant Pangu transformed and created the world. Primordial union has been reestablished, and the practitioner partakes of the unlimited supply of original, primordial, ever-circulating *qi*.

This oneness with the universal flow of *qi* is further actualized in the practice of *qi*-absorption through active visualization. While the breath is being held, practitioners move the *qi* actively through the body, making sure it flows equally to all parts. The *Yangxing yan-ming lu* says:

> Visualize the body clearly: head, face, nine orifices, five or-gans, four limbs, even the tips of the hairs. All has to be present. Become aware of the *qi* as a cloud circulating in the body, rising up to the nose and mouth and descending to the tips of the ten fingers. This will lead to purity and harmony, and a perfect spirit. (2.1b)

The *Fuqi jingyi lun* describes this slightly differently:

> First, visualize the *qi* in the lungs for some time, then feel it run along the shoulders and into the arms, until it reaches your hands that have been curled into fists. After this visu-alize it gently moving down from the lungs and into the stomach and spleen area, from where it moves into the kid-neys. Allow it to flow through the thighs and into the legs and feet. You will know that you are doing it right when you feel a slight tingling between skin and flesh, sort of like the crawling of tiny insects. (7b)

In either case, adepts should see and feel the *qi* as it moves through the body, guided consciously by intention. The word used for "visual-ize" is *cun* 存, which literally means "to be," "to be present," "to exist." In this sense it is also used to denote extreme longevity, as in the fa-mous passage in the *Zhuangzi*, where Guangchengzi exclaims: "I alone survive!" (ch 11). In Daoist practice, the word is used in its causative mode, in the sense of "to cause to exist" or "to make pre-sent." It thus means that the meditator by an act of conscious concen-tration and focused intention causes certain energies to be present in certain parts of the body or makes specific deities or scriptures ap-pear before his or her mental eye. For this reason, the word is most commonly rendered "to visualize" or, as a noun, "visualization." Since, however, the basic meaning of *cun* is not just to see or be aware of but to be actually present, the translation "to actualize" or "actualization" might at times be more correct. In other words, practitioners guide the *qi* throughout the body, making it actively present in all its parts, thus again reinforcing the connection to universal power and purity.

The Five Sprouts

This same intense connection is also activated in another variant of the absorption of *qi*, the practice of the Five Sprouts (*wuya* 五芽). Known from early Highest Clarity materials, this serves the cosmicization of the body through the ingestion of the energies of the five directions and is also known as the "method of mist absorption" (Robinet 1989, 165-66). The practice begins with swallowing the saliva while chanting invocations to the original *qi* of the four directions. As adepts next face the direction, they visualize its *qi* in its appropriate color. A vague haze at first, the *qi* gradually forms into a round ball, and then is condensed into a pill. As such adepts ingest the sprout and guide it mentally to its appropriate organ. Over time the adept's body is pervaded by cosmic *qi* and transformed into a vehicle of universal energies.

The incantations are short and to the point. As the *Fuqi jingyi lun* says:

> Green Sprout of the East:
> Be absorbed to feed my [internal] green sprout [liver].
> I drink you through the Morning Flower [upper teeth].
>
> Vermilion Elixir of the South:
> Be absorbed to feed my [internal] vermilion elixir [heart].
> I drink you through the Elixir Lake [lower teeth].
>
> Lofty Great Mountain of the Center:
> Be absorbed to feed my [internal] essence and qi.
> I drink you through the Sweet Spring [molars].
>
> Radiant Stone of the West:
> Be absorbed to feed my [internal] radiant stone [lungs].
> I drink you through the Numinous Liquid [lip saliva].
>
> Mysterious Sap of the North:
> Be absorbed to feed my [internal] mysterious sap [kidneys].
> I drink you through the Jade Sweetness [tongue saliva].
> (3ab)

In each case, the text also specifies that adepts should pass the tongue along a certain part of the lips and teeth, matching the incantation. They should then lick the lips, rinse the mouth by filling it with saliva, and swallow. It is to be repeated three times for each sprout. The practice is also described in the *Taishang yangsheng taixi qi jing* 太上養生胎息氣經 (Highest Qi Scripture on Nourishing Life Through Embryo Respiration, DZ 819), which adds:

> Always practice the *qi* methods at midnight, at the *zi* or *yin* hour. Stand upright, dressed in proper cap and gown. Activate your golden bridge [tongue] and waken the jade radiance [breath] to balance the flowery pond [mouth]. Rinse with the sweet spring [saliva] and numinous fluids. Contract your nose and make the *qi* return, going up to the head and sinking down inside the mouth. There it can transform into jade spring [refined saliva]. From here, pull the *qi* to the root of the tongue, swallow, and send it off.

> As you do all this, there should be a rumbling sound in both your throat and your abdomen. As you guide the *qi* into the elixir field, it is like a child just born and already able to cry. This is called the root of long life. When hungry, eat the *qi* of spontaneity; when thirsty, drink the juice of the flowery pond. Then you can be forever full and satiated. (3b-4a)

Undertaken over a prolonged period, this technique eventually creates a spirit embryo (*lingtai* 靈胎) inside the practitioner, a supernatural alter ego that is able to draw in the primordial *qi* of the universe and is directly nourished by it. "This method of absorbing *qi* involves visualizing the heart as if it contained a baby in the mother's womb. After ten months it is complete, tendons and bones are harmonized and supple" (*Taixi jing* 1a). The spirit embryo develops as and when the practitioner reconnects with his spirit root (*linggen* 靈根), the last remnant of the connection the individual had with the universe while in the womb and often identified with the tongue, thus explaining the extensive tongue movements of the practice.

The spirit embryo therefore grows from the same root as the physical body of the practitioner, but is connected closely with primordial creation. Once the spirit embryo is sufficiently developed, the practitioner becomes one with it and his or her consciousness merges into it. The adept transforms into a spirit immortal.

The worldview of the Five Sprouts technique is complex. There is no simple appreciation of the Dao and the world. Rather, the world is divided into phases, directions, and times. This creates a spherical appreciation of the universe best understood as relating to the eight trigrams (*bagua* 八掛) of the *Yijing* 易經 (Book of Changes; see Wilhelm 1950). Fuxi, an early culture hero of the Chinese, delineated time and direction through the trigrams. They accord with the directions of the compass in their postnatal arrangement, as well as in a spherical alignment which relates back to the primordial egg of the cosmic creator Pangu.

In the prenatal alignment, the seven directions of the sphere (up, down, front, back, right, left, center) are conjoined with the eighth: time. The latter is related to the shifting of these reference points as the observer moves and rotates. Shifting is only possible with the conception of time. The method of the Five Sprouts attempts to recreate the egg structure of the universe of Pangu by performing the technique at the proper time and facing the proper direction.

Yet the five phases are also included. Practitioners attempt to draw them into themselves and, through accordance with time and the directions of the trigrams, hope to reshape their bodies back into the primordial egg. If successful, they will be permeated with the essence of the five phases so that the meeting ground in the center of their

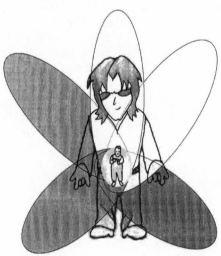

bodies becomes a microcosm of the Dao and allows the development of the spirit embryo. The practitioners' digestive systems and therefore their postnatal *qi* remain active, though elevated and able to ingest the sprouts of the phases. This is in many ways parallel to the technique of *shiqi*, but it is utterly different in that the body is no longer a mechanism of breathing and digestion but has become a microcosm of the universe (see Fig. 5).

Fig. 5: Fusion of the Five Sprouts creates the embryo

From the East Asian medical standpoint, the *xie* components of the person's body are corrected, not by expelling them but by embracing them in their entirety. By effectively dissolving the distinction between the self and the universe through Five Sprouts practice, the person's body becomes as integrally whole as the universe itself. There is no distinction of *xie* and *zheng* in the greater universe, and the practitioner becomes "big" enough to enjoy the same state. Having done so, the spirit embryo forms in the womb of the microcosmic universe of the practitioner's body. The embryo is *zheng* with the *qi* of the universe, and the implication is that the physical and nonphysical worlds are concomitant but separate. The practitioner carries an embryo but is not pregnant; he is the universe but remains himself.

This is radically different from the technique of enclosing the *qi*. While enclosure is an act of sympathetic magic, the absorption of the sprouts is an act of thaumaturgy, i.e, a magical technique of summoning elemental forces to shape the world to the will of the practitioner. By conjuring and invoking the essence of the phases, the mechanics of the body are altered so that the practitioner has effectively bred a familiar—a spirit that can be made present at will, induced to inhabit the person, and serves at one's beck and call. However, this familiar is not an alien or other entity, but the practitioner's own *qi* in conjunction with that of the universe. A further purpose of the embryo is to become a house for the practitioner's consciousness and thus to allow him to join the spiritual bureaucracy of the immortals. This carries with it the physical death of the practitioner, but leads to spiritual life in a perfected state. The view here is transcendent. There is salvation from the fate of decay through the transformation of *qi* into pure spirit.

Conclusion

The absorption of *qi*, in method and concept, is radically different from the technique of eating *qi*. Absorption leads to being permeated by cosmic *qi* and transformed into an integral aspect of the universe. The individual *xie* nature is reoriented to be *zheng* in alignment with the whole. This model has no transcendent salvation, but proposes an immanent return to the primordial state, which is forever there but never accessed. Here lies a fundamental difference of Chinese medicine and Western and Indian concepts of religion. Rather than attempting to find salvation by transcendence and separation from the world, the practitioner of this methodology transforms the world by reorienting himself within it. Aligned perfectly with the whole, the mechanics of the body are restructured to match the greater workings of all things, and practitioners are no longer scavengers in the phenomenal world who eat and defecate. Rather, they are as intact a part of the system as the rivers and mountains. They are one with the Dao, and thus infinitely fulfilled.

As Daoism continued to evolve, the various techniques of *qi* manipulation and transformation were joined and integrated in various ways, reflecting different worldviews and conceptualizations of the religion as they combined into a unified system. In the middle ages, however, the practices were still separate and the absorption of *qi* was clearly distinct from the practice of eating *qi*.

From the early texts we can thus understand the practices more clearly. While eating *qi* utilizes the digestive system and replaces foodstuffs with a more rarefied substance, the absorption of *qi* leads to a complete permeation by *qi*. The practitioner is pervaded by the *qi* to the point that he or she is transformed by it. This also matches the original terms. "Eating" has the implication of nourishment, ingestion, and defecation, while "absorption" is not done with foodstuffs, but with medicine. The implication is that one will not be nourished by the medicine, which is digested and its waste defecated, but that one will be permeated and transformed by it. This is the key to appreciating the difference between eating and absorbing *qi*. Eating *qi* is simple replacement, while absorbing *qi* aims to transform the mechanism of the practitioner's body into something more than mere human, retooling the inner mechanics of the body's subtle components and thus leading the practitioner to immortality.

Bibliography

Bensky, Dan, and Andrew Gamble. 1986. *Chinese Herbal Medicine Materia Medica.* Seattle: Eastland Press.

Eckman, Peter. 1996. *In the Footsteps of the Yellow Emperor: Tracing the History of Traditional Acupuncture.* San Francisco: Cypress Books.

Engelhardt, Ute. 1987. *Die klassische Tradition der Qi-Übungen. Eine Darstellung anhand des Tang-zeitlichen Textes Fuqi jingyi lun von Sima Chengzhen.* Wiesbaden: Franz Steiner.

_____. 1989. *"Qi* for Life: Longevity in the Tang." In *Taoist Meditation and Longevity Techniques,* edited by Livia Kohn, 263-94. Ann Arbor: University of Michigan, Center for Chinese Studies Publications.

Harper, Donald. 1998. *Early Chinese Medical Manuscripts: The Mawangdui Medical Manuscripts.* London: Wellcome Asian Medical Monographs.

Jackowicz, Stephen. 2003. "The Mechanics of Spirit: An Examination of the Absorption of *Qi.*" Ph. D. Diss., Boston University, Boston.

Kohn, Livia, ed. 1989. *Taoist Meditation and Longevity Techniques.* Ann Arbor: University of Michigan, Center for Chinese Studies.

Maspero, Henri. 1981. *Taoism and Chinese Religion.* Translated by Frank Kierman. Amherst: University of Massachusetts Press.

Mitamura, Keiko. 2002. "Daoist Hand Signs and Buddhist Mudras." In *Daoist Identity: History, Lineage, and Ritual,* edited by Livia Kohn and Harold D. Roth, 235-55. Honolulu: University of Hawaii Press.

Mugitani Kunio. 1987. "Yōsei enmei roku kunchi." *Report of the Study Group on Traditional Chinese Longevity Techniques,* no. 3. Tokyo: Mombushō.

Needham, Joseph, et al. 2000. *Science and Civilisation in China* Vol. VI.6. Medicine. Edited by Nathan Sivin. Cambridge: Cambridge University Press.

Ni, Maoshing. 1995. *The Yellow Emperor's Classic of Medicine.* Boston: Shambhala.

Porket, Manfred. 1974. *The Theoretical Foundations of Chinese Medicine*. Cambridge, Mass.: MIT Press.

Robinet, Isabelle. 1989. "Visualization and Ecstatic Flight in Shangqing Taoism." In *Taoist Meditation and Longevity Techniques*, edited by Livia Kohn, 157-90. Ann Arbor: University of Michigan, Center for Chinese Studies Publications.

Sivin, Nathan. 1988. *Traditional Medicine in Contemporary China*. Ann Arbor: University of Michigan, Center for Chinese Studies.

Switkin, Walter. 1987. *Immortality: A Taoist Text of Macrobiotics*. San Francisco: H. S. Dakin Company.

Unschuld, Paul. 1985. *Medicine in China: A History of Ideas.* Berkeley: University of California Press.

Wilhelm, Richard. 1950. *The I Ching or Book of Changes*. Princeton: Princeton University Press, Bollingen Series XIX.

Wiseman, Nigel, and Ken Boss. 1990. *A Glossary of Chinese Medical Terms and Acupuncture Points*. Brookline, Mass.: Paradigm.

Wu, Nelson, and Andrew Wu. 1999. *The Yellow Emperor's Canon of Internal Medicine*. Beijing: China Science and Technology Press.

Zhang, Yuanming. 1996. *Secret of Immortality from the Holy Mountains of China*. Los Angeles: Institute of Traditional Science and Culture Publishing.

Chapter Four

Life Without Grains:

Bigu and the Daoist Body

Shawn Arthur

Throughout history, Daoists have paid great attention to issues of the body and have developed many sophisticated ways of refining its internal workings through the manipulation of *qi*. Besides breathing, healing exercises, sexual control, and Qigong, the observance of specialized dietary regimens has formed an important practice of Daoist body cultivation for the past two millennia.

Dietary regimens include the avoidance of meat and alcohol as well as of the so-called five strong vegetables (*wuxin* 五辛; onions, scallions, leeks, garlic, and ginger) for physical and ritual purification. They also involve shorter or longer periods of fasting and replacing food intake with pure *qi* for the attainment of long life and an ethereal spirit body. Fasting in particular is known as *bigu* 辟穀, literally "avoiding grains," which seems to be the term's original intention.[1] However, since the general Chinese diet was based on rice and other staples, avoiding grains by extrapolation came to mean abstaining from eating large amounts of, or even any, ordinary foodstuffs. In other words, *bigu* indicated the avoidance of all food as much as the modern compound *chifan* 吃飯, "to eat rice," means to have a meal.

Before the Tang dynasty (618-907), practitioners usually fasted for short periods as part of ritual purification, while long-term *bigu* prac-

---

[1] Several other terms express the same basic idea as *bigu* and are used interchangeably in the literature. They include *duangu* 斷穀 ("to cut off grains"), *quegu* 却穀 ("to eliminate grains"), *xiuliang* 休粮 ("to cease cereals"), and *jueli* 絕粒 ("to abandon staples").

tice did not avoid but merely limited food intake. Ideally combined with other cultivation methods, *bigu* meant to ingest small amounts of regular food plus a variety of herbal concoctions (including appe-tite-suppressing herbs), alcoholic herbal infusions, and cosmic *qi* sup-plements. However, ideological changes in the Tang and Song dynas-ties produced a significantly different and more austere type of *bigu*, one that included no foods whatsoever and focused more predomi-nantly on the ingestion of cosmic *qi* to supplement the body's needs.

Today, practitioners utilize *bigu* in conjunction with other cultivation techniques both to increase their health and as an initial stage of in-ner alchemy. They begin their *bigu* regimen with the ingestion of small amounts of herbs to help the body acclimate to not eating ordi-nary foods and culminate their practices with long periods of com-plete fasting supplemented by *qi* ingestion. In the following, I will outline the main aspects and developments of *bigu* in the history of Daoism, presenting textual evidence, expectations of *bigu* practices, and a variety of techniques and recipes together with observations and explanations by contemporary practitioners.

Earliest Evidence

Daoist dietary theory derives largely from the ancient Chinese pen-chant for pursuing longevity that dates back to the Western Zhou (1112-771 B.C.E.), when it is mentioned on bronze vessels and in po-ems of the *Shijing* 詩經 (Book of Odes). By the fourth century B.C.E. the desire for long life had led not only to the initiation of a Chinese medical tradition but also to the quest for physical immortality—a pursuit which became central to the development of Daoism—either through natural medications, alchemically created gold, or the super-natural elixirs of the immortals who lived on the mythical isles of Penglai 蓬萊 in the Eastern Sea (see Yü 1964).

The oldest textual evidence that provides an early medical viewpoint about the physical body is found in the Warring States period (479-221 B.C.E.), in the *Zuozhuan* 左傳 (Master Zuo's Commentary). It de-scribes the cause of illness in terms of excesses of the six atmospheric forms of *qi*, i.e., shady yin, sunny yang, wind, rain, dark, and light. Further discussions of the body, its vital functions, and techniques for cultivating and preserving life appear in later texts of this period, such as the "Neiye" 內業 (Inward Training) chapter of the *Guanzi* 管子 (Book of Master Guan; see Roth 1999). The latter contains the most coherent example of early Chinese longevity practices, resting on a foundation of Chinese cosmology as associated with the philosopher Zou Yan 鄒衍 of the late fourth century B.C.E., which proposes a complex correspondence system linking the cosmos, society, and human beings through yin-yang and the five phases.

The "Neiye" is "a collection of rhymed verses on the nature of the cosmos, the nature and activity of the mind, and the practice of several related methods of mental and physical self-discipline aimed at physical health, longevity, and self-transcendence" (Roth 1991, 611). It explains that all aspects of the cosmos are manifestations of Dao, the ultimate cosmic principle, and that meditation is a form of heart-mind (*xin* 心) training that helps attunement to Dao. Awareness of the movements and patterns of *qi* and the manipulation and purification of internal energies are of paramount importance. The text includes the first instance of dietary practice as part of a cultivation regimen. It says that, in order to maintain inner harmony, one should neither eat too much nor eat too little:

> For all the Way of eating is that:
> Overfilling yourself with food will impair your vital energy
> And cause your body to deteriorate.
> Overrestricting consumption causes the bones to wither
> And the blood to congeal.
> The mean between overfilling and overrestricting:
> This is called "harmonious completion."
> (16.4b7-8; Roth 1999, 90)

Another early mention appears in the *Zhuangzi* 莊子 (Book of Master Zhuang, DZ 670; see Graham 1981; Watson 1968), which alludes to various kinds of people seeking long life, such as the 1,200-year old Guangchengzi 廣成子 (ch. 11; see Legge 1962, 299). A classic passage that also refers to diet describes the spirit men (*shenren* 神人) of Mount Gushi, whose flesh and skin were like ice and snow and whose manners were as delicate as those of young women. Maspero has:

> (1) They do not eat the five [grains];
> (2) they breathe the wind and drink the dew;
> (3) riding upon clouds and air and driving flying dragons,
>   they journey beyond the Four Seas;
> (4) when their spirit is concentrated, it causes creatures not
>   to be attacked by pestilences and grains to ripen every
>   year. (1981, 416-17)

This is one of the first mentions of the "five grains," commonly identified as rice, millet, wheat, oats, and beans, and a standard phrase in later description of Daoist dietary practices. However, the *Zhuangzi* does not specify the practices any further, since it was critical of people who followed popular self-cultivation regimens such as breath cultivation and healing exercises (Harper 1998, 115; Legge 1962, 364). Still, the note indicates that people practiced such methods in the third century B.C.E.

A fuller presentation of self-cultivation practices appears in a collection of medical manuscripts discovered in a tomb at Mawangdui 馬王堆 in the Hunan province, dated to 168 B.C.E. Unlike the *Zhuangzi*, which idealized cultivation of the spirit and shunned the limitations of bodily matters, the Mawangdui manuscripts present a broad interest in macrobiotic hygiene, medicine, as well as exorcistic and shamanic methods of self-cultivation. Donald Harper identifies four main branches of macrobiotic hygiene, including breath cultivation, physical exercises, sexual cultivation, and dietetics (1998, 126-27; see also Engelhardt 2000).

With regard to diet practices, the most important manuscript is *Quegu shiqi* 却穀食氣 (Eliminating Grain and Eating *Qi*), an early example of the grain avoidance practices of southern shamans in conjunction with Zou Yan's fourth century cosmological theories that relate grains to Earth (square) and *qi* to Heaven (round) (Harper 1998, 159). The text discusses grain avoidance through the consumption of the herb tongue-fern (*shiwei* 石韋; *Pyrrosia lingua*) combined with a regular regimen of morning and evening breathing exercises. The latter change with the seasons and include six types of *qi* that should be inhaled or ingested and five types of atmospheric *qi* to be avoided (Harper 1998, 25).

Other Mawangdui manuscripts describe methods to avoid grains, to supplement food with the ingestion of *qi* through respiration and visualization, and to replace ordinary nourishment with herbs and alcoholic infusions. For example, the *Shiwen* 十問 (Ten Questions) argues that pine (*song* 松), arbor-vitae (*mubai* 木白; *Thuja orientalis*; a.k.a. white cypress), and tongue-fern are the best replacements for grains during a grain-elimination regimen in order to combat the symptoms of heavy-headedness, lightness of the feet, and itchiness that are associated with such a process (Harper 1998, 131). Overall, the earliest evidence shows that dietary practices were firmly part of medical and longevity traditions and were commonly undertaken among aristocrats with access to training and sufficient leisure.

Visions of Immortality

Beyond the medical and long life traditions, in the Former Han dynasty (206-6 B.C.E.), dietary methods increasingly came to be associated with the quest for magical powers and immortality. An important group striving for such powers was the *fangshi* 方士 or "occult technicians." The term has been variously translated as "gentlemen possessing magical recipes," "occultists," "magicians," "necromancers," "Masters of Esoterica," "masters of method," and literally "recipe masters" (see DeWoskin 1983; Ngo 1976; Raz 2004). I prefer "occult technicians" because the expression combines the complexity of the original term and focuses on the esoteric nature of the practitioners' knowledge and their secretive methods of transmission.

These *fangshi* were marginal figures in established Han society. Engaged in techniques of physical and spiritual control, they had their minds set on interaction with the spirit world and in the process of their training acquired magical powers. They could predict fortunes and perform astrological divinations, analyze weather patterns and make rain, heal diseases and exorcise demons, communicate with the dead and conjure up spirits, advise on military strategy and provide magical weaponry (DeWoskin 1983, 23-35). Like the medical specialists of the time, they "shared a common interest in understanding natural phenomena and their consequences for humankind" (Harper 1998, 10, 44).

If willing to serve as ritual specialists or guides to long life, the *fangshi* were occasionally also employed in the Han civil service, where they were classified as astronomers, yin-yang specialists, diviners, and interpreters of *qi*-patterns. However, the *fangshi* also practiced herbalism, incantations, and early forms of alchemy. Through their efforts as well as through those of longevity seekers and mountain hermits, immortality gradually emerged as a practical vision, combining the thoughts and techniques of early seekers, occult technicians, Huang-Lao Daoists, proponents of natural philosophy, correlative cosmologists, shamans, and medical specialists (see Puett 2004).

A key document in this context is the *Huainanzi* 淮南子 (Book of the Prince of Huainan, DZ 1184; see Le Blanc 1985; Roth 1992), compiled under the sponsorship of Liu An 劉安 (179-122 B.C.E.), the Prince of Huainan. Interested in all matters of the occult, he gathered together several thousand *fangshi*, Huang-Lao Daoists, and scholars, encouraged their practices, and had them compile a text explaining and integrating a wide range of ideologies on cosmology, astrology, self-cultivation, medicine, and immortality (see Major 1993).

The *Huainanzi* presents a comprehensive and organized cosmological view based on the concept of resonance (*ganying* 感應). Resonance is the idea that the different aspects and levels of the cosmos are synchronically linked and engage in constant energetic interaction. It informs personal actions, explains the evolution of the biological and mineral worlds, and develops the theory that the macrocosm can be recreated on a microcosmic scale.

Resonance theory asserts that once people identify the relationship between two or more aspects of the cosmos (whether ideological, spiritual, or physical), they can then influence their interaction or attune their bodily energies to them (see Le Blanc 1992). Based on the cosmology of yin-yang and the five phases, it links human morality to cosmic processes and human virtues as well as social regulations to cosmic norms (Sivin 1995, 27-28). As a result, people's spontaneous actions—based on their human nature—ideally change consistently to reflect both the *qi* ("energy") and the *li* 理 ("natural pattern," "principle") of any particular season and situation (Kohn 2004, 13).

Resonance and its corresponding concepts were instrumental not only to the creation of complex self-cultivation regimens followed by later Daoists but also to the development of Chinese alchemy. Alchemy in this context can be defined as the combination of taking macrobiotic or cinnabar elixirs (*dan* 丹) and the chemical synthesis of gold to attain an immortal body (see Pregadio 2000). Its earliest form appeared as the ingestion of natural gold, based on the idea that physical immortality could be attained by emulating the unchanging quality and eternal power of gold, thereby developing a cosmic resonance with it. To become like gold, people ingested food and drink served on plates and cups made from purified gold through a process called "projection," whereby a small quantity of alchemically transformed gold would change any other metal into "gold."

According to Joseph Needham, these magically transformed artificial gold vessels could also function as "containers for the elixir substances of vegetable origin, the herbs of deathlessness" (1974, 13). If adepts did not become spirit immortals through this process, they could at least reach physical longevity. Once they attained long lives, they could aspire to meet immortals to receive an immortality drug or to alchemically create their own elixir.

Although many metals used in elixir recipes—such as arsenic, cinna-bar powder, mercury, lead, and tin—are highly toxic, cultivation practitioners desired some of the effects produced by their ingestion. Many texts on alchemical immortality claim that an elixir regimen changed adepts' awareness of their physiology in positive ways. Ad-epts felt less hungry, lighter in their bodies, healthier, and more vig-orous (at least for a time). They had stronger libidos and a greater sense of well-being. It is also possible that some elixir ingredients im-proved people's health by curing diseases, removing parasites, raising iron levels in the blood, counter-acting malnutrition, and curing im-potence (Needham 1974, 282, 285, 293-94). Also, long-term ingestion of these elixirs may well have caused hallucinations of ecstatic flights, spirit visions, and superhuman powers.[2]

People who practiced these various dietary and alchemical techniques appear in the *Liexian zhuan* 列仙傳 (Immortals' Biographies, DZ 294), a collection of seventy legendary immortals' biographies ascribed to Liu Xiang 劉向 (77-6 B.C.E.). About half of the figures attained immor-tality by ingesting gold elixirs or lesser drugs such as cinnabar dust, cinnamon, fungus, mica, pine fruit, ginseng, scallions, Angelica root, and peaches (Needham 1976, 9; Akahori 1989, 76).

For example, the first immortal of the collection is Chisongzi 赤松子 or Master Redpine who became immortal because he avoided grains, practiced healing exercises, and did regular deep breathing (Kalten-mark 1953, 35). Another famous figure who attained immortality through dietary means is Maonü 毛女, the Hairy Lady (see Fig. 1). Her biography says:

> Maonü, also known as Jade Mistress, has been seen by hunters on Mount Hua for several generations. Her body is covered with hair. She claims that she was among the pal-ace ladies of the First Emperor and first fled to the moun-tain during the troubles that attended the downfall of the Qin dynasty.

> There she encountered the Daoist recluse Guchun, who taught her how to live on pine needles. As a result of this diet, she became immune from cold and hunger, and her body became so light that it seemed to fly. For over 170

---

[2] Evidence indicates that Daoists and alchemists used hallucinogenic smoke, such as marijuana, in their incense burners and took the hallucino-genic mushroom fly-agaric, *Amanita muscaria*, as well as cacti and fungi that had similar psychedelic effects (Needham 1974, 116, 122, 150).

years the mountain grotto where she makes her home has resounded with the thrumming of her zither. (Kaltenmark 1953, 160)

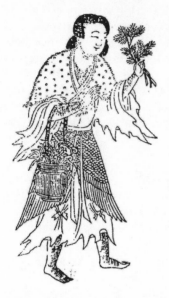

Unlike earlier practitioners, whose ideals were worldly in orientation and who focused primarily on increasing longevity, adepts in the *Liexian zhuan* strove to develop a spirit body that would transcend the mortal world and would allow them to reside among other immortals and to enjoy the pleasures of the paradises (Yü 1964, 89; Needham 1974, 80). They used herbs, plants, and elixirs, as well as *qi*-cultivation and virtuous actions to attain their goals.

As Daoists became organized into communal groups in the Later Han dynasty (9-220 C.E.), longevity and immortality practices were further standardized and began to merge with devotional activities.

Fig. 1: Maonü, the Hairy Lady.

For example, the *Taiping jing* 太平經 (Scripture of Great Peace, DZ 1101; see Hendrischke 2000) of the second century combines previously documented cultivation practices with religious aspects of Daoism, merging them with prayers and sacrifices, talismans and incantations, as well as with Confucian social philosophy which prescribed specific ethics and virtues and prohibited abandoning the family to search for immortality (Needham 1974, 126). About the abstention from grains it says: "If you desire to know the meaning of the child in the womb, then do not eat for ten months, and then the spirits will communicate with you" (ch. 52). As Hu Fuchen notes, this directly continues earlier forms of "obtaining immortality and supernatural powers by means of *bigu*" (2004, 385).

The major focus of the *Taiping jing*, however, was the idea that the preservation and prolongation of life was the highest virtue of Heaven and Earth and that the different kinds of spirits and human beings had to work together smoothly and harmoniously to create Great Peace. Each had to maintain their *qi* at utmost harmony, so that it could flow perfectly and create prosperity, long life, and good fortune. In concrete terms this meant that members of the organization ob-

served strict moral rules and participated in various communal cere-
monies. They had to eat moderately, to abstain from alcohol, to undergo medical healing, to harmonize their minds with music, and to
practice meditations (Kaltenmark 1979, 41-44). Immortality, and
thereby the practice of dietary regimens, had advanced from a personalized individual pursuit to the overarching goal of a Daoist community and, by extension, the world at large.

The World of Ge Hong

While some Daoists organized themselves into communities and expanded the ideals and practices of immortality, individuals still continued to become hermits and to seek ultimate realization for themselves through self-cultivation and alchemical means. The most important works on this aspect of early Daoist food cultivation are the
Baopuzi 抱朴子 (Book of the Master Who Embraces Simplicity,
DZ1185; trl. Ware 1966) and the *Shenxian zhuan* 神仙傳 (Lives of the
Spirit Immortals; trl. Campany 2002) written by the government official and would-be alchemist Ge Hong 葛洪 (287-347) (see Fig. 2).

Born as a southern aristocrat in a small town near Jiankang 建康
(modern Nanjing 南京), he was inspired by his *fangshi* uncle Ge Xuan
葛玄 (ca. 164-244) and developed a strong interest for otherworldly

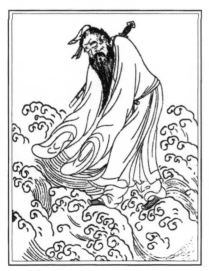

pursuits. At the age of fourteen,
he became a disciple of the hermit
and alchemist Zheng Yin 鄭隱,
then married and was further
influenced by his father-in-law
Bao Jing 鮑靚, another cultivation
practitioner. After serving the
imperial administration in various minor capacities, Ge Hong
resigned his position to study
longevity and immortality full
time (Pregadio 2000, 167). He
wandered around the country in
search of ancient manuscripts
and learned masters, then came
home to write down his findings.

Fig.2: Ge Hong.

In his autobiography—the first of its kind in Chinese literature—Ge Hong describes how he eschewed official positions and even avoided social interaction with his peers because his one aim in life was to become immortal, i.e., to reach a state of perfect health and extended longevity that would allow the concoction of an alchemical elixir and ascension to the heavens. For Ge Hong, immortality was reached not so much through religious observances, such as prayers and rituals, although he certainly believed in the magical efficacy of talismans and incantations.

Rather, for him the desired state could be attained by laying a groundwork of long life attained through longevity techniques—healing exercises, breathing, special diets, and meditations—followed by the great alchemical endeavor, which had to be undertaken in secrecy in the seclusion of the mountains and required numerous costly ingredients and holy scriptures, transmitted either by the gods in trance sessions or by hermit masters after the passing of strictly-guarded texts (Kohn 1991, 85-86). Although he never compounded any elixir by the time he compiled his writings, hagiographic accounts suggest that he retired to Mount Luofu 羅浮山 late in life to devote himself to preparing the great elixir (Ware 1966, 6-21).

Ge Hong's *Baopuzi* contains various dietary prescriptions using mushrooms, fruits, alcoholic infusions, and elixirs, all purported to facilitate *bigu* practices with limited intake. It mentions numerous herbs and minerals, meant to aid in the quest for immortality, that are divided into three categories: elixirs (generally based on cinnabar), spirit drugs (generally in the form of mountain fungi), and common herbal or food substances. On the practice of *bigu*, he says:

> To avoid bringing about suffering, it is best not to cut off grain [intake] but merely to regulate the diet, which you can do with a hundred different methods. Sometimes, after you have taken a few dozen pills of mineral-based medicine to protect the [body's] interior, you can withdraw [to a secluded mountain] for forty or fifty days without hunger.

> Refined pine [*song* 松] and cypress [*bai* 柏] as well as thistle [*shu* 术; *Atractylodes macrocephala*] can also protect the interior, but they are inferior to the great medicine. In the end, they will not last more than ten years, while at the same time either you will be able to abstain [from food] for 100 or 200 days or you must daily ingest the ingredients to reach a state of no appetite.

> At other times, fine foods are prepared and consumed to ut-
> ter satiation, and then medicines are taken to nurture the
> things that have been eaten, so that they will not be di-
> gested, and you will be able to abstain [from food] for three
> years. (ch. 15; see Ware 1966, 244)

Ge Hong asserts that the practice of fasting brings about various
positive results, including weight loss, removal of intestinal worms,
elimination of hunger and thirst, calming of the heart-mind, reversion of the hair from white to black, the renewed growth of lost teeth,
increase in vitality and overall stamina, improvement in eyesight and
hearing, concentration and refinement of internal energies, stabiliza-
tion of the circulation of *qi*, cleansing of the viscera by elimination of
built-up wastes in the body, and changes to the physical digestive
system that make it redundant.

Ge Hong also discusses in detail how to ingest herbs, how to locate
them by traveling into the mountain wilderness with the help of protective talismans, and how to find those spirit fungi (*lingzhi* 靈芝; ex-
crescences) that are only visible to the most astute and purified seekers and only if they wear magic talismans on their belt for protection
from malevolent forest entities and for raising awareness of positive
nature spirits. At specific times of the year, in certain places, many of
the 600 different fungi are visible as rocks, vegetation, and small
creatures to adepts who have practiced *bigu* for an extended length of
time, have attained a certain degree of insight and awareness, and
who possess the correct talismans. As Ge Hong writes:

> If you desire to seek excrescences and herbs, entrance into
> the famous mountains must be done either during the third
> or ninth moons, since these are the months when the moun-
> tains are open and produce the divine medicines. Refrain
> from going on days when the mountains are hostile. . . .
>
> It is essential to wear a belt with the Numinous Treasure
> talismans, have a white dog on a leash, and carry a white
> chicken. If a peck of white salt and an Open the Mountain
> talisman are placed on a large rock, and a bunch of Wu hops
> is held as you enter the mountain, the gods of the mountain
> will be pleased and you will certainly find excrescences. (ch.
> 11; see Ware 1966, 185-6)

Once picked, these fungi are proclaimed to provide the adept with a range of powers including the abilities to fly, to see in the dark, to become invisible, and to prolong life for thousands of years.[3]

Another important effect of dietary practices for Ge Hong was the removal of the so-called Three Worms (*sanchong* 三蟲) or Three Corpses (*sanshi* 三尸), divine parasites that reported misdeeds to the celestial administration and, upon orders from above, proceeded to make the body sick and weak. The Three Worms were originally organic parasites like leeches that, as Wang Chong 王充 (ca. 127-200) says in his *Lunheng* 論衡 (Balanced Discussions), "live in the marshes beneath the soil and gnaw their way through the feet of people, just as the Three Worms gnaw through their intestines" (16.3; Forke 1962, 2:363). To get rid of them, certain herbal decoctions were ingested. For example, the biography of the famous physician Hua Tuo 華托 in the *Sanguo zhi* 三國志 (Record of the Three Kingdoms) says:

> To expel the Three Worms, use a green pasty powder made from the leaves of the lacquer tree. Take it for a long time, and the Three Worms will be expelled, the five inner organs will be greatly strengthened, the body will feel light, and there will be no white hair. (ch. 29; see DeWoskin 1983)

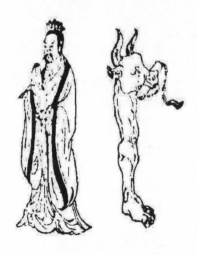

Ge Hong expands this notion. No more mere "leeches" gnawing on human intestines, the Three Worms became the Three Corpses (see Fig. 3), officials of the celestial administration who reside in the body—side by side with more positive body gods—to monitor human behavior and to punish sins and transgressions. A mixture of parasites, demons, and souls, they reside in the head, torso, and lower body of the individual and there, assisted by a group of lesser gnawers known as the Nine Worms, do all they can to incite the person to do evil and fall ill.

Fig. 3: The Upper and Lower Corpses.

---

[3] See also Penny's discussion of the immortals' powers (2000, 125-6).

After the death of the host, when the souls proper have been sent off to suffer in the hells and to be prepared for rebirth, they remain with the corpse and gorge themselves on its flesh.

Having partaken of the human body, they are then able to assume its former intact shape and to appear as ghosts, feasting further on the offerings laid out for the dead. Thus they have a vested interest in bringing a person to death quickly and without mercy. The *Baopuzi* describes them:

> There are Three Corpses in our bodies. The Three Corpses are made of matter, yet they are not fully corporeal: they are real like heavenly souls (*hun* 魂), numinous powers, ghosts, and spirits. They desire to cause people to die early, at which time these Corpses are able to act as ghosts, to move around freely, and to partake of people's sacrifices and libations.
>
> On every *gengshen* 庚申 day [the 57th day of the 60-day cycle], they ascend to heaven [and report on] the way each person behaves to the Director of Destiny. Similarly during the last night of the moon [cycle], the Stove God makes a journey to heaven [to report on] our criminal behaviors. For the more important misdeeds, three hundred days are deducted from our lives. For lesser sins, three days are removed. (ch. 6; see Ware 1966, 115-16)

According to Ge Hong and later Daoist belief, the human body consists of many energies and entities among which the Three Corpses are the most destructive that actively hasten our decay. Normal nourishment, especially grains and bloody foods, keep these demonic parasites alive. As long as they are alive, moreover, they hold the body rooted firmly to the earthly realm and prevent any refinement of internal energies or attainment of immortality—the stated main goal of early Daoist practice.

In accordance with the heightened powers of the Three Corpses, they can no longer be expelled by the mere concoction of crude herbs but require ritual measures, ethical purity, and stronger medicines. Thus:

> Ingesting pure unadulterated lacquer causes people to enter into communication with the gods and to attain long life. Mix ten pieces of large crab into [the lacquer] and dissolve this in mica water or jade water. Ingest this and the Nine Parasites will altogether drop from you, and impure blood will flow out by way of nosebleeds. (ch. 11; see Ware 1966, 190)

Ingesting such herbal and chemical substances during a grain avoidance dietary regimen not only helps to kill the Three Corpses, but
also accentuates the body's more subtle energies, thus further facilitating their refinement. Once the body is sufficiently purified, a variety of gods, who naturally inhabit it but leave when they are sub-
jected to impurities through immoral actions, negative emotions, and
strongly flavored foods, will again take up residence in the interior
palaces and will assist in the preparation of the body for immortality.
Only then can adepts concoct the Great Elixir, perfect their health,
and attain magical powers. As Ge Hong says about a concoction of
realgar, earthworm excreta, and cinnabar pounded into a paste and
fired extensively:

> If you take one pill the size of a small bean three times daily
> until one pound (*jin* 斤) has been consumed, the Three
> Worms and Concealed Corpses and the hundred illnesses
> will all flee [your body].

> If blind, you will see. If deaf, you will hear. If old, you will
> again feel as if you were thirty years old. Entering fire you
> will not be burned. The hundred evils, the many poisons, as
> well as all cold, wind, heat, and dampness no longer will be
> able to encroach upon you.

> Once you have taken three pounds [using this method], you
> will be able to walk on water. The hundred gods of the
> mountains and streams will come to serve and protect you.
> Your life will last as long as that of nature itself! (ch. 16; see
> Ware 1966, 275-76)

Adepts in this mode of Daoist dietary practice therefore abstain from
grains but replace their normal nourishment with alchemically refined substances that may be more or less poisonous but have the effect of transforming the body both physically and spiritually and can
only be concocted and taken in a formal ritual setting that requires
careful preparation, utmost seclusion, and complete secrecy. Although
Ge Hong disagreed in most cases with the idea that ingestion of
herbal substances can confer immortality, as Daoism continued to
develop, valorization of alchemical elixirs waned and they were replaced with less poisonous herbs and fungi.

The *Wufuxu*

In the wake of Ge Hong, the most detailed outline of medieval dietary practices appeared in the *Taishang Lingbao wufu xu* 太上靈寶五符序 (The Highest Explanation of the Five Numinous Treasure Talismans, DZ 388; hereafter cited as *Wufuxu*). Like the *Baopuzi* it is a collection and explanation of methods to increase longevity and to attain immortality. The text began as a single scroll written in the Later Han dynasty by *fangshi* or immortality seekers from the Shandong area in eastern China, was edited in the third century by Ge Hong's uncle Ge Xuan in the Jiangnan region near modern Nanjing, and by the fifth century had grown into a three-scroll text—the form in which it has survived in the Daoist canon (see Yamada 1989, 113; 2000, 238; Eskildsen 1998, 54; Raz 2004). The final redaction seems to have been performed by Ge Hong's great grandson Ge Chaofu 葛巢甫, the founder of the Numinous Treasure (Lingbao 靈寶) school of southern aristocratic Daoism in the late fourth and early fifth centuries (see Bokenkamp 1983; Yamada 2000).[4]

The *Wufuxu* presents an important synthesis of ideas and compiles many ascetic dietary regimens. In many ways it represents a culmination of thinking about the body, immortality ideas, and food intake that did not substantially change until inner alchemy (*neidan* 內丹) began to emerge several centuries later—and even then the dietary regimen was not so much changed as it was refined to include a heightened sense of Buddhist-inspired ethics and a change in the conception of immortality from physical to spiritual.[5]

Especially the second chapter of the text contains a list of seventy longevity and immortality recipes that are all but one based on plant or animal materials (see Fig. 4). Sixteen recipes contain sesame (*huma* 胡麻; *Sesamum indicum*), thirty-two are herb-infused alcohols,

---

[4] There are many similarities between Ge Hong's *Baopuzi* and the *Wufuxu* (see Raz 2004). Evidence indicates that Ge Hong's writings were informed by and early edition of the *Wufuxu*.

[5] Neidan practices abandoned the ideal of maintaining the physical body indefinitely in favor of refining the *shen* 神 (spirit) component of the body, using alchemical metaphors and extensive visualization practices rather than ingesting elixirs and cultivating an immortal embryo that combines the refined *shen* and consciousness of the Daoist (see Needham 1974, 1976; Penny 2000; Pregadio 2000).

and others use various fungi and vegetable materials including: China root fungus (*fuling* 茯苓; *Poria cocos*; a.k.a. Tuckahoe), pine tree sap, locust tree parts (*huaimu* 槐木; *Sophora japonica*), lotus parts (such as the fruit: *lianshi* 蓮實; *Nelumbo nucifera*), variegated dry land root (*zhanglu* 章陸; *Phytolacca acinosa*; a.k.a. poke root), earth yellow herb (*dihuang* 地黃; *Rehmannia glutinosa* Liboosch), yellow essence (*huangjing* 黃精; *polygonatum sibiricum*; a.k.a. Solomon seal), and asparagus root (*tianmendong* 天門冬; *Asparagus cochinchinensis*). For example, the "Recipe of the Perfected for Cutting Off Grain" states:

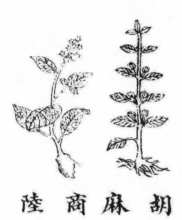

Obtain two pecks [*dou* 斗] of the "Great Vanquisher" [*jusheng* 巨勝; sesame] and five pints [*sheng* 升] of large red peppers [*jiao* 椒]. Discard the black shells of the sesame seeds. When finished, mix and pound the two items and then strain them.

At the beginning ingest five portions daily with three bowls of broth until none is left. Also, you can sweeten the dose with honey. Ingest a portion the size of a small chicken egg four times daily.

Fig. 4. Poke Root and Sesame

Gradually and naturally, you will not be hungry even in famine. Also, you can ingest it plain. This medicine will give the ability to abstain from grains. If you thirst, only drink water; do not eat anything else. If you eat other things, you will again hunger. You will be able to increase your energy potential a hundredfold. Cold and heat will not encroach upon you. The hundred illnesses will entirely be healed. Spirit immortality will be the natural result. (2.5b-6a)

This recipe exemplifies the largest problem that a translator encounters when approaching a Daoist recipe text: the drug names are often metaphorical or symbolic and are extremely difficult to correlate to the physical materials. Reasons for this are many, including that drugs often had different names in different regions and that drug names evolved over time. Also, Daoist names which refer to the spiritual qualities of the herbs were unknown by the compilers of *materia medica* texts, the imprecise nature of naming led to several natural referents obtaining a single name, and substitute ingredients occasionally took on the names of the original ingredient which they replaced.[6] The *Wufuxu* contains many ingredients whose accurate identification is questionable; however the name for sesame in this recipe, "Great Vanquisher," is cross-referenced in an earlier recipe with its more well-known name *huma* 胡麻,"Barbarian Hemp."

The "Recipe of the Perfected for Cutting Off Grain" also introduces the idea that *bigu* practices in the *Wufuxu* do not necessarily indicate the avoidance of all food. Here one begins the regimen with three small meals of the ground sesame-pepper mix and broth, then gradually decreases this to four small daily portions. The recipe not only indicates that sesame-based *bigu* facilitates healing, but it seems as though this drug also has hunger-suppressing qualities, as does the following recipe for "Causing People to Not Grow Old, to Have a Long Life, to Expel the Three Worms, to Cure the Hundred Illnesses, and to Make Poisons Unable to Injure People." It says:

> Take thirty pounds [*jin* 斤] of Variegated Dry Land Root [poke root] that was gathered on the first, second, ninth, tenth, eleventh, or twelfth month. The root gathered during other months is not useful.
>
> Take it and cleanse and wash it. Coarsely slice it into lengths of two to ten inches [*cun* 寸]. Do not allow it to be exposed to wind. In a thin silk bag place it all to hang in the northern part of your room for sixty days. The shade-dried powder can be prepared by sifting one *cun* of the recipe into seven parts water.
>
> Ingest once daily before eating or drinking. After ten days you will see spirit beings. After sixteen days you will be able to send these spirit beings to obtain gold, silver, and valuables and to create a room that has all that you desire. After eighty days you will be able to see as far as a thousand miles. After a hundred days your body will be able to travel by flying, mounting the winds, and walking among the clouds. Your intestines will change into muscles. After ingesting this for a long time, you will become an immortal. (2.11ab)

According to Stephen Eskildsen, "poke root is a toxic plant commonly used as a diuretic. Its toxicity may have been what made it an effec-

---

6 See *Shiyao erya* 石藥爾雅 (Commentary on [the Names of] Minerals and Herbs, DZ 901); Harper 1998, 100.

tive hunger suppressant. ... The poke root's poison affected the body rapidly and drastically. Apparently it made the adept eat less because the poison caused an inflammation in the intestines" (1998, 60-1). Furthermore, poke root seems to have a hallucinatory effect in that it can help one communicate with gods and other spirit beings and is also associated with expelling the Three Corpses.

This long life recipe also introduces another important aspect of Daoist drug therapies: the integrated use of cosmological correlations ideology and resonance theory. Many recipes in medieval texts directly relate the herbs to idealized properties associated with yin and yang, the five phases, and the *qi* associated with different times of the year. Thus the recipe demands that poke root should be harvested during the cooler winter or yin and spring or lesser yang months and dried in a yin environment before use. The idea of correlations regarding properties of medicinal drugs is at least as old as the Mawangdui manuscripts where "there are examples of choosing drugs and applying therapy that reflect theoretical considerations, including: plants picked at the summer solstice or eggs collected in spring, which are understood to have solar, yang potency (prior magico-religious belief regarding the solar virtues of drugs must also be taken into account); homeopathy; and environmental factors affecting treatment" (Harper 1998, 90-91).

The next recipe represents an important genre of medicinal prescriptions: the four-ingredient recipe. There are many four-part recipes in Daoist medical and immortality literature, as this continues to be a common form of Chinese medical prescription. One herb is the major active ingredient; another serves to supplement the major herb or to affect secondary symptoms; and the remaining two balance the major two ingredients by counteracting adverse side-effects, enhancing the desired effects, and/or mitigating the potency of the main herbs. "The Four Substances for Immortality Recipe As Received By the Yellow Emperor from Yellow Lightness" explains:

> The first is called Extensive Radiance [*hongguang* 鴻光].
> The second is called A Thousand Autumns [*qianqiu* 千秋].
> The third is called The Ten Thousand Ages [*wansui* 萬歲].
> The fourth is called Compassion Ink Seeds [*cimoshi* 慈墨實].
>
> Mix together these four things to make a pill. Use white pine [*baisong* 白松] sap [to make pieces] as large as a chicken egg. Ingest this for seven years. Your body will live 43,000 years and will not die. After a long time of ingesting

it, you will be able to share in heaven's and earth's mutual protection.

The Yellow Emperor [Huangdi 黃帝] asked: "The appearance of these four things looks like what? Could I please hear about that?" Huang Qing said: "Extensive Radiance is Mother of the Clouds [*yunmu* 雲母; mica]. A Thousand Autumns is Curly Cedar [*juanbo* 卷栢].

They grow between mountain rocks. Ten Thousand Ages is Marsh Drainage [*zexie* 澤瀉; *Alisma orientalis*; a.k.a. Oriental water plantain]. Compassion Ink is Edible Greens' Fruit [*xianshi* 莧實; *Amaranthus mangastanus*; a.k.a. pigweed]. Make a pill by means of pine tree sap [*songzhi* 松脂] the size of a chicken egg. In the morning and in the evening ingest one pill. This will allow you to lengthen your existence while not having hunger or thirst." (2.14b-15a)

Here again is evidence of differing nomenclature for naming medicinal ingredients. The first set of names represents the Daoist "mystical" names, and the later set represents more well-known names. In fact, this recipe is still used by Daoists and some Chinese medical doctors today. The properties of this recipe are founded upon the mica's medicinal properties, which are beneficial for the stomach and for counteracting the diabetes-like symptoms of the Chinese medical diagnosis of *tangniao bing* 糖尿病 (Sweet Urine Sickness).

Also, it seems that drugs for the stomach could be quite useful for facilitating a successful fasting regimen. Regarding mica, Ge Hong writes: "Other things decay when buried and burn when placed into fire; however when the five micas are placed into a raging fire, they do not burn at all even after a long time, and they are not corrupted or destroyed even after a long burial. Therefore they are able to confer long life" (ch. 11; see Ware 1966, 187). This is a good example of why some materials are chosen, such as evergreen products and certain minerals: they have perceived properties—such as permanence or greenness throughout the winter months—which through correlation and resonance can be directly associated with the intended results of dietary regimens and self-cultivation therapies.

Another interesting facet of the recipes in the *Wufuxu* is the range of physical and spiritual benefits that *bigu* regimens afford the practitioner. For example, "A Recipe for Extending the Years and Increasing Longevity" says:

> Place ripe locust tree seeds [*huaizi* 槐子] in a cow's intestine
> [*niuchang* 牛腸], and put this in a dark place to dry for a
> hundred days. After that, swallow one piece with your meal
> in the morning and evening. After ten days your body will
> lighten. After thirty days your white hair will revert to
> black. After one hundred days your face will become radiant.
> After two hundred days, a galloping horse will not be able to
> keep up with you. (2.16a-b)

Many recipes in the *Wufuxu* attribute similar health-related properties to immortality recipes: as adepts progress in their ascetic dietary
regimens their bodies "lighten"[7], white hairs return to a black color,
lost teeth grow back, complexions brighten, hearing and sight improve, *qi* becomes stronger, and stamina increases.

Besides these detailed herbal and mineral recipes, the *Wufuxu* also
presents practices of ingesting the Five *Qi* and absorbing lunar and
solar essences. For example, to absorb the essence of the sun, practitioners must

> concentrate on the sun and visualize a small child dressed
> in red in your heart. His garments are embroidered in the
> five colors and he emits a bright red radiance. Massage
> yourself with both hands from the face down to the heart;
> repeat this twelve times. You will see the red radiance of
> the sun and a yellow energy will appear before your eyes.
> Make this enter your mouth and swallow it twice nine times.
> Then rub your heart and recite an incantation. (1.18b; Ya-
> mada 1989, 119)

In this practice, adepts eat the *qi* (*shiqi* 食氣) of the sun to nourish
their bodies and to enhance their cosmic connection. Toshiaki Yamada argues that this is not a dietary practice since its theoretical
foundation involves beliefs about deities in the human body and the
use of ritual incantations (1989, 112, 119). However, I find that in the
fifth century Daoists actively combined grain avoidance diets and *qi*
eating practices into a mutually reaffirming regimen that gradually
replaced normal foodstuffs with cosmic *qi* absorption.

Zhang Xingfa argues that *qi* ingestion is actually one of the five types
of *bigu* practice for health and purification that also include cutting
down on food intake, avoiding processed food, eliminating fat and salt

---

[7] It is unclear whether this quality refers to severe weight loss, a
psychological (maybe hallucinogenic) feeling of lightness that comes from not
eating ordinary foods, or a side-effect of the medicine.

from the diet, and utilizing medicinal herbs to supplement a fasting regimen (2003, 288). According to him, *bigu* means to abstain from the five grains and various other foods, but does not involve the complete cessation of food intake—if all food is avoided, *qi* will still need to be ingested. This contention matches the fact that the *bigu* regimens in the *Wufuxu* utilize *shiqi* techniques to purify the body to such an extent that the practitioner is able to connect with cosmic deities and body gods.

The spiritual aspect of *bigu* practice is reflected in the developmental pattern on which many of the *Wufuxu* recipes are based: first the adept uses herbal supplements to bolster health, to decrease food intake, to reduce hunger, to fortify *qi*, and to eliminate the Three Corpses. After a few months or years, depending upon the recipe, the ideal physical body will be attained—complete with increased stamina and a youthful appearance.

The second major effect includes supernatural powers such as extreme longevity and the abilities to fly, to disappear, to run faster than a horse, and to transform one's physical shape. Evidently these powers are meant as signs that practitioners are progressing in their *bigu* practice as they do not represent an end in and of themselves. The last stage of *bigu* practice is marked by a stronger and more manifest connection to the spiritual realm: the practitioner will meet earthly and cosmic spirits, the myriad body gods will take up residence, and immortality of the physical body will eventually be attained.

Modern Versions

With the evolution of Daoism in the Tang (618-907) and Song (960-1279) dynasties came further development of the cultivation of internal bodily processes through complex visualizations of the internal processes of the body and their correlation to cosmological phenomena and the many gods within the body who control its internal processes.

The development of inner alchemy overshadowed the earlier creation of chemical elixirs and became the sole focus of many Daoists. For example, inner alchemy practices became one of the main forms of self-cultivation in the Complete Perfection (Quanzhen 全真) school, founded by Wang Chongyang 王重陽 (1112-1170) in 1167 in Shandong—the same area that brought forth many *fangshi* a thousand years earlier. Regarding food intake, the Quanzhen school mandates specific dietary restrictions for all members in order to avoid impurity of the body and mind. Louis Komjathy notes, "The Quanzhen hagiographies mention various types of physical austerities. It seems that begging and restriction of food intake were general commitments among most, if not all, of the early adepts" (2005, 183).

Ma Danyang 馬丹陽 (1123-1183), a student and successor of Wang Chongyang, in the seventh of Ten Admonitions in his *Zhenxian yulu* 真仙語錄 (Recorded Sayings of Perfected Immortals, DZ 1256) tells followers to "be cautious in speech, controlled in food and drink, and moderate in taking rich flavors. Discard luxury and give up all love and hate [for sensory pleasures]" (1.8b-9b; Komjathy 2005, 170). Part of the reason for this precept is to help the adept avoid the Four Hindrances of alcohol, sex, wealth, and anger, which Wang explains in the *Chongyang quanzhen ji* 重陽全真集 (Chongyang's Anthology on Complete Perfection, DZ 1153) will have myriad harmful influences such as obscuring the adepts' innate nature, retarding spiritual development, injuring the body's *qi*, dissipating virtue, and decreasing longevity (1.18a-19a; Komjathy 2005, 166).

Complete Perfection followers use *bigu* regimens to prepare for important rituals and, according to contemporary Daoist priests, employ it as a first step for serious internal cultivation regimens such as inner alchemy (Pregadio 2000, 482). Dietetics for them is part of a wide-ranging ascetic discipline meant to fulfill the body's physical and spiritual potentials by cleansing impurities, opening mystical body locations, circulating and refining subtle energies, and awakening divine capacities. As Komjathy explains: "The Quanzhen adept, quite literally, actualized a different kind of body, within which something different circulated," and "asceticism was seen as foundational for health and well-being" (2005, 182; also Eskildsen 2004, 39-94).

Inner alchemy represents an evolution in Daoist thinking about alchemy and immortality, especially regarding insights into the physical body. In the middle ages, adepts created interior refinement through materials of the natural world, such as herbs and minerals. Inner alchemists, on the other hand, refined their energies from within their own bodies. The earlier concern for longevity and the transformation of the physical body changed to a focus on developing a spiritual body that consisted of rarified *qi, shen*, and consciousness. This higher self would eventually emerge during meditation with the abilities to travel throughout the cosmos and to continue to exist even after death.

Building upon earlier explanations of the body's internal functioning, inner alchemy practitioners argued that *bigu* practice should lead to avoiding all foodstuffs, because as internal energies were refined, the body felt reduced craving and requirement for "mundane" sources of nutrition and sooner or later found support sustenance in pure *qi* acquired through visualization and meditation. In other words, the prolonged practice of inner alchemy by way of ingesting *qi* necessitated the practice of grain and food avoidance and represented a change in the meaning of *bigu* from avoiding grains and diminishing food intake to avoiding all food ingestion.

The contemporary use of *bigu* represents the culmination of almost two and a half millennia discussing the demerits of ingesting grains and general foodstuffs and the preference for self-cultivation and other religious aims. Although Western science indicates that prolonged fasting will hasten death, there are many Daoists in China today who have succeeded in going without food for weeks or months. My first introduction to Complete Perfection Daoists in Sichuan indicated that *bigu* practice is a dead art. No one I met would admit to attempting the methods or knowing someone who had. However, after persevering in my research and talking with many Daoists about the history of and ideas behind the elusive *bigu* practice, I came into contact with some—both monastics and householders—who had practiced *bigu* regimens for durations of two to six months.

My most cogent informer was Professor Hu Fuchen 胡孚琛 (b. 1945) of the Chinese Academy of Social Sciences in Beijing. Although Hu had studied with several wandering Daoists over twenty years, his training as a scientist made him skeptical of the practice. In the 1990s, however, he was diagnosed with multiple serious diseases and, as a last resort, decided to practice *bigu* as a complete fasting regimen.

He developed a daily Qigong routine and undertook extensive fasts. Now, ten years later, his illnesses are either completely gone or in remission, and he still practices *bigu* every spring for four to eight weeks. He also wrote a detailed log of his practices and activities which indicates that people can indeed live and increase their health through long periods of fasting, supplemented with small amounts of fruit for the first few weeks and with cosmic *qi* for the duration of the fast.

Professor Hu confirms the earlier Daoist contention that the initial weight loss during the first month of *bigu* practice is followed by weight gain although no food is eaten. The body loses its equilibrium during the beginning phase, but increases in functioning and gains weight when it finds a new balance. At the same time, health dramatically improves, hearing and sight sharpen, and stamina and well-being increase. As a result of his personal experiences, Professor Hu today actively advocates the renewed activation of Daoism to make it more accessible to contemporary practitioners and interpret its methods in modern terms (Hu 2002, 2005).

The *Bigu* System

How, then, does the practice work as a coherent system? What are some of the typical methods, stages, and experiences?

First of all, not all Daoists practiced *bigu* in the same way. Given the caveat that *bigu* is one part of a larger, more complex regimen for self-cultivation, practitioners' choice of dietary practice depends upon their training and goals. For example, there are different general dietary restrictions for ascetic and hermitic Daoists who work toward immortality, Daoist monastic community members, and laity. Thus practicing *bigu* for ritual preparation and performance generally only requires three to five days of fasting. Also, many Daoist schools insist on fasting before receiving and studying important scriptures.

Practicing with the goals of improving health and longevity requires longer fasts, i.e., weeks or months, and a regular repetition as, for example, annually, to provide optimal benefits. The practitioner often can eat small amounts of food or herbal supplements and still drink small amounts of water. Beyond all these, there are some fasts for immortality that prohibit the ingestion of all foodstuffs and which can last much longer, even for years. Thus, for example, inner alchemy training requires long-term practice for at least ten months in order to create and gestate the immortal embryo.

Based on this, the first effort required in any *bigu* regimen is deciding upon one's goal and setting a limit for how long one will practice. According to contemporary practitioners, this is an important step as the actual decision aids the practitioner's mental state of preparation.[8] The second most important preliminary effort is working on improving one's health, *qi*-flow, and awareness of personal *qi*. Although adherents claim that *bigu* practices improve health, eyesight, hearing, and so on, it is necessary to do preparatory *qi*-work to attain

---

[8] Personal correspondence and interviews in Beijing and Chengdu, China, September-December, 2004.

a heightened inner awareness. Daoist long life and leisure practices—meditations, Qigong, Taiji quan, music, and calligraphy—all explicitly work to refine *qi*. Preparatory dietary practices such as avoiding too much food and strong spices, while ingesting herbs to bolster internal *qi*, are also recommended.

Bigu preparation makes the adept's life more quiet, relaxed, and stable so as to avoid upsetting the body's delicate system of *qi* flow. During a *bigu* regimen, practitioners should also remain in a relatively calm life situation because as they refine their *qi*, acute sensitivity to environmental *qi* patterns (of both harmony and chaos) develops and can interfere with their practices. This is one reason why Daoist texts advocate that serious self-cultivation practitioners should remove themselves from society and live in a secluded, secret place for the duration of the practice.

However, some contemporary Daoists and *bigu* practitioners do not leave the world in order to practice. Their argument is that the best hermits are able to hide themselves within society and do not flee to the mountains. They also say that, with proper preparation and sufficient focus of will, living in the world should not be a problem, although one has to take care to avoid too much "contact with commoners or, worse, disbelievers which may upset preparation" (Akahori 1998, 85).

After one has found a place to practice, one undergoes ritual purification. The *Baopuzi* suggests a hundred-day purification regimen of bathing in herbal-infused water, concentration exercises to clear the mind, and abstaining from any polluting foods as well as activities, thoughts, and objects (ch. 4; see Ware 1966, 75). To be successful in a *bigu* endeavor, the practitioner must be completely dedicated to the practice and must develop the proper mental attitude. With these preparations, as my informants indicated, the body's desire for regular foods naturally diminishes to such a degree that long-term *bigu* practice is not particularly difficult.

Once preparation is complete, the ascetic dietary regimen begins by gradually decreasing regular food intake while supplementing the diet with herbs and medicines. In contrast to short-term fasts, such as three-day purifications for ritual purposes, when the dramatic stoppage of food (coupled with meditations, chanting, and lack of sleep) elicits particular psychological responses and a sudden heightened awareness, for long-term fasts adepts alter their food intake over several weeks. They begin to ingest supplemental herbs, fruit, and/or medications as transitional foods, allowing their body to gradually acclimate to the ingestion of cosmic *qi*.[9]

Even then the first steps of *bigu* practice are usually frought with difficulty. Already Ge Hong points out that "a moment of crisis generally occurs at an early stage when medicines are being taken and starches abandoned, and it is only after forty days of progressive weakening, as one uses only holy water and feeds solely on breath, that one regains strength" (ch. 15; Ware 1966, 247). Similarly Henri Maspero notes that

> this very severe diet was not without painful moments. Without grains and meat any practitioners is undernourished, and Daoist authors admit that at the beginning one may have numerous troubles, some of them general (vertigo, weakness, sleepiness, difficulties in moving), others local (diarrhea, constipation, and so on) (1981, 335).

Although the fasting regimen begins gradually, the body undergoes stress and weakening. There will be significant weight loss because of the lack of normal dietary intake. To counteract these problems, practitioners continue to follow special breathing methods. Also, negative effects usually lessen after a few weeks and health benefits begin to appear.

Adepts also typically experience a range of psychological symptoms, such as hallucinations from lack of food, side effects from herbal concoctions, visions from accompanying meditations, or imaginings resulting from auto-suggestions and the intentional focus on immortal's images. Experiences may include feelings of lightness, cleanliness, and purity; a perception of perfected health; a heightened awareness of Dao and other important cosmic energies including the gods; the feeling of a radical separation from reliance on social foodstuffs and thus from ties to society; and a sense that one is able to fly. Also, fasting often increases sensitivity to *qi* and allows it to flow more smoothly. Furthermore, many adepts experience the ability to heal others by aligning or infusing their *qi* into the body of a patient. Evidently, liver and heart *qi* are particularly useful for providing this curative effect (Eskildsen 1998, 48; Hu 2004).

---

[9] The conclusion of long-term *bigu* practice is another gradual process whereby the adept carefully reintroduces water, lard, teas, and herbal soups to re-lubricate the unused digestive tract (see *Baopuzi*, ch. 15; Ware 1966, 244-45).

The final set of experiences attained by *bigu* practitioners relates to their perception of spiritual accomplishment and development. The range of spiritual experiences include: an awareness of and harmony with Dao and the ceaselessly changing cosmic energies; the meeting of and conversation with body gods, cosmic deities, and immortals; the installation of deities within the purified body; an awareness of and conversing with worldly spirits, such as spirit mushrooms; and the removing of one's strongest connection to the earthly realm through the Three Corpses. Later Daoists also found benefits to their inner alchemical practices from the practice of *bigu*, because the practice facilitated the development of the immortal embryo in the lower cinnabar field.

All of these experiences indicate that *bigu* practitioners are progressing toward their ultimate goal of immortality. They also provide evidence about Daoist conceptions of immortality and the body. For example, in the ideology of immortality seekers, the physical body, once sufficiently purified, transforms into an immortal body and thus is not connected to the earthly realm. This idea appears in the many professed experiences of lightness of the body and flying abilities. Through building on extant concepts of cosmological correlation and its relationships to the body, as well as explanations and techniques provided by the unfolding medical tradition and Daoist religious views, immortality seeking Daoists have utilized, and still do practice, *bigu* to great benefit to themselves and subsequently to the reaffirmation of their beliefs.

Conclusion

Self-cultivation practices were present in China long before the emergence of Daoism as a codified religion, and these regimens along with theories of resonance-based cosmological correlation informed the development of both Daoism and Chinese medicine, which utilize dietary practices to meet their goals. In fact, Daoists have made grain and food abstention dietary practices an integral aspect of their spiritual cultivation regimens.

Bigu regimens originally limited an adept's food intake while supplementing with a variety of herbal substances and cosmic *qi*; yet as Daoist ideals evolved, *bigu* techniques also evolved into the more austere practice of ingesting *qi* while completely abstaining from all physical foodstuffs. Furthermore, although early Daoist texts such as the *Baopuzi* and *Wufuxu* indicate that *bigu* practice should continue indefinitely until such time as immortality is attained, contemporary Daoists perform periodic shorter-term *bigu* regimens—from a few days to a year—to pursue their various goals.

Contemporary adepts practice *bigu* in conjunction with other *qi* cultivation techniques with the goal of improving health, purifying the body, and initiating inner alchemy training. As they begin their *bigu* regimens, they eat small amounts of herbs—such as those presented in the various recipes of the *Wufuxu*—to help their bodies acclimate to ingesting cosmic *qi* in lieu of ordinary foods. As potential side-effects wane, practitioners can wean themselves off of herbal supplements and claim to be able to rely only on *qi* ingestion for their bodies' needs. It is at this point that the Daoist goal of creating an immortal spiritual body can be pursued.

According to Western medical science, a dietary regimen that involves not eating for a prolonged period of time is extremely dangerous and medically impossible. In contrast to this contention, Chinese sources have chronicled 2,400 years of practitioners who have utilized ascetic dietary regimens and self-cultivation practices in the pursuit of health and longevity. According to ancient texts and contemporary Daoist testimonies alike, humans may not be able to thrive by eating only grains and breads, but man can exist on *qi* alone.

Bibliography

Akahori Akira. 1989. "Drug Taking and Immortality." In *Taoist Meditation and Longevity Techniques*, edited by Livia Kohn, 71-96. Ann Arbor: University of Michigan, Center for Chinese Studies Publications.

Bokenkamp, Stephen. 1983. "Sources of the Ling-pao Scriptures." In *Tantric and Taoist Studies*, edited by Michel Strickmann, 2:434-86. Brussels: Institut Belge des Hautes Etudes Chinoises.

Campany, Robert F. 2002. *To Live As Long As Heaven and Earth: A Translation and Study of Ge Hong's Traditions of Divine Transcendents*. Berkeley: University of California Press.

DeWoskin, Kenneth J. 1983. *Doctors, Diviners, and Magicians of Ancient China*. New York: Columbia University Press.

Engelhardt, Ute. 2000. "Longevity Techniques and Chinese Medicine." In *Daoism Handbook*, edited by Livia Kohn, 74-108. Leiden: E. Brill.

Eskildsen, Stephen. 1998. *Asceticism in Early Taoist Religion*. Albany: State University of New York Press.

_____. 2004. *The Teachings and Practices of the Early Quanzhen Taoist Masters*. Albany: State University of New York Press.

Forke, Alfred. 1972. *Lun-Heng: Wang Ch'ung's Essays*. New York: Paragon.

Graham, A. C. 1981. *Chuang-tzu: The Seven Inner Chapters* and Other Writings from the Book of *Chuang-tzu*. London: Allan & Unwin.

Harper, Donald. 1998. *Early Chinese Medical Manuscripts: The Mawangdui Medical Manuscripts*. London: Wellcome Asian Medical Monographs.

Hendrischke, Barbara. 2000. "Early Daoist Movements." In *Daoism Handbook*, edited by Livia Kohn, 134-64. Leiden: E. Brill.

Hu Fuchen 胡孚琛. 2002. "21 Shiji de xindaoxue wenhua zhanlue 21 世纪的新道学文化战略" in *Zhongwai zhexue de bijiao yu rongtong* 中外哲学的比较与融通, edited by Chang Yuyou 场与有, ch.6. Beijing: Zhongguo shehui kexue chubanshe.

_____ and Lü Xichen 吕锡琛. 2004. Daoxue tonglun: Daojia, Daojiao, Dandao 道学通论： 道家，道教，丹道. Beijing: Shehui kexue wenxian chubanshe.

_____. 2005. "21st Century Strategies for New-Daoism." Translated by Shawn Arthur and Chen Xia. The Empty Vessel: A Journal of Daoist Philosophy and Practice, 12.4: 36-44.

Kaltenmark, Max. 1953. *Le Lie-Sien Tchouan*. Beijing: Université de Paris.

_____. 1979. "The Ideology of the *T'ai-p'ing-ching*." In *Facets of Taoism*, edited by Holmes Welch and Anna Seidel, 19-52. New Haven: Yale University Press.

Kohn, Livia. 1991. *Taoist Mystical Philosophy: The Scripture of Western Ascension*. Albany: State University of New York Press.

_____. 2001. *Daoism and Chinese Culture*. Cambridge, Mass.: Three Pines Press.

_____. 2004. *Cosmos and Community: The Ethical Dimension of Daoism*. Cambridge, Mass.: Three Pines Press.

Komjathy, Louis. 2005. *Cultivating Perfection: Mysticism and Self-Transformation in Early Quanzhen Daoism*. Ph.D. Dissertation, Boston University.

Le Blanc, Charles. 1985. *Huai-nan-tzu: Philosophical Synthesis in Early Han Thought*. Hong Kong: Hong Kong University Press.

_____. 1992. "Resonance: Une interpretation chinoise de la realite." In *Mythe et philosophie a l'aube de la Chine imperial: Etudes sur le Huainan zi*, edited by Charles Le Blanc and Remi Mathieu, 91-111. Montréal: Les Presses de l'Université de Montréal.

Legge, James. 1962. *The Sacred Books of China: The Texts of Taoism*. New York: Dover.

Li Yanwen 李衍文, ed. 2003. *Zhonghua yaoyinming cidian* 中草药异名词典. Beijing: Renmin weisheng chubanshe.

Major, John S. 1993. *Heaven and Earth in Early Han Thought: Chapters Three, Four, and Five of the Huainanzi*. Albany: State University of New York Press.

Maspero, Henri. 1981. *Taoism and Chinese Religion*. Translated by Frank Kierman. Amherst: University of Massachusetts Press.

Needham, Joseph, et al. 1974. *Science and Civilisation in China*, vol. V.2: Spagyrical Discovery and Invention—Magistries of Gold and Immortality. Cambridge: Cambridge University Press.

_____. 1976. Science and Civilisation in China: vol. V.3: Spagyrical Discovery and Invention: Historical Survey, from Cinnabar Elixir to Synthetic Insulin. Cambridge: Cambridge University Press.

Ngo, Van Xuyet. 1976. *Divination, magie et politique dans la Chine ancienne*. Paris: Presses Universitaires de France.

Penny, Benjamin. 2000. "Immortality and Transcendence." In *Daoism Handbook*, edited by Livia Kohn, 109-33. Leiden: E. Brill.

Pregadio, Fabrizio. 2000. "Elixirs and Alchemy." In *Daoism Handbook*, edited by Livia Kohn, 165-95. Leiden: E. Brill.

Raz, Gil. 2004. "Creation of Tradition: the Five Talismans of Numinous Treasure and the Formation of Early Daoism." Ph.D. Dissertation, University of Indiana at Bloomington.

Roth, Harold D. 1991. "Psychology and Self-Cultivation in Early Tao-istic Thought." *Harvard Journal of Asiatic Studies* 51: 599-650.

_____. 1992. *The Textual History of the Huai-Nan Tzu.* Ann Arbor: Association of Asian Studies Mon+ograph.

_____. 1999. *Original Tao: Inward Training and the Foundations of Taoist Mysticism.* New York: Columbia University Press.

Shen Liansheng 沈连生. 2004. Bencao gangmu 本草纲目. Beijing: Huaxia chubanshe.

Sivin, Nathan. 1995. "State, Cosmos, and Body in the Last Three Centuries B.C." Harvard Journal of Asiatic Studies 55: 5-37.

Skar, Lowell and Fabrizio Pregadio. 2000. "Inner Alchemy (*Neidan*)." In *Daoism Handbook*, edited by Livia Kohn, 464-97. Leiden: E. Brill.

Ware, James R. 1966. *Alchemy, Medicine and Religion in the China of AD 320.* Cambridge, Mass.: MIT Press.

Watson, Burton. 1968. *The Complete Works of Chuang-tzu.* New York: Columbia University Press.

Yamada, Toshiaki. 1989. "Longevity Techniques and the Compilation of the *Lingbao wufuxu.*" In *Taoist Meditation and Longevity Techniques*, edited by Livia Kohn, 97-122. Ann Arbor: University of Michigan, Center for Chinese Studies Publications.

_____. 2000. "The Lingbao School." In *Daoism Handbook*, edited by Livia Kohn, 225-55. Leiden: E. Brill.

Yü, Ying-shih. 1964. "Life and Immortality in the Mind of Han-China." *Harvard Journal of Asiatic Studies* 25: 80-122.

Zhang Xingfa 张兴发. 2003. *Daojiao neidan xiulian* 道教內丹修炼. Beijing: Zongjiao wenhua chubanshe.

Chapter Five

Yoga and Daoyin

LIVIA KOHN

Yoga, the eight-limb system associated with Patañjali's *Yogasūtras*, and Daoyin, the Daoist practice of guiding (*dao* 導) the *qi* and stretching (*yin* 引) the body, at first glance have a lot in common. They both focus on the body as the main vehicle of attainment; they both see health and spiritual transformation as one continuum leading to perfection or self-realization; and they both work intensely and consciously with the breath. In both Yoga and Daoyin, moreover—unlike in Taiji quan and the majority of Qigong forms—physical stretches and movements are executed in all the different positions of the body, while standing, moving, sitting, and lying down. Postures are often sequenced into integrated flows and named either descriptively or after various animals.

In both systems, too, practitioners follow certain basic ethical rules and guidelines for daily living, geared to create an environment best suited to personal transformation. They learn the exact way to execute postures and movements, they gain awareness and control of their respiration, and they work to adjust the breath in accordance with the body postures. Adepts moreover use the strengthening of the muscles, loosening of the joints, and awareness of internal energies to enter into states of absorption and deeper meditation, relating actively to spiritual powers and seeking higher levels of self-realization.

Does that mean, then, that Yoga and Daoyin represent essentially the same system, just expressed in Indian and Chinese forms? Do they pursue the same goal, use the same methods, and reach similar stages, just formulated in different languages and terminologies? Is there, maybe, even an historical overlap, a mutual influence between the two systems that might explain their closeness? Or are the similarities coincidental—predicated upon the fact that all bodies move and stretch and breathe and that certain exercises are essentially good for us—and mask a deeper layer of complex and sophisticated differences in worldview, history, social role, and practice?

To answer these questions, I will look at the philosophical foundations of both practices, at historical origins and sociological settings, at their developments over time, and at the way they relate healing to spiritual realizations. I conclude with a look at their concrete practices and a general evaluation of their similarities and differences.

Philosophical Foundations

The body in Yoga forms an integral part of a body-mind continuum that cannot be separated and is seen as one. This continuum is one aspect of the material world ground, known as *prakṛti*. *Prakṛti* is real and eternal, dynamic and creative, inert and primordial (Eliade 1969, 31). It is the underlying substance of all that exists, the "noumenal matrix of creation," "the realm of the multitudinous phenomena of contingent existence" (Feuerstein 1980, 29). It lies deep underneath the surface of natural everyday reality, representing its ultimate ground and creative potential, yet it is also the concrete, material world as it exists with all its different forms, modes, and transformations. *Prakṛti* at the root of all being is not accessible by ordinary sensory means but can be reached through yogic introspection after long periods of training and meditative immersion.

So far, *prakṛti* sounds amazingly like Dao. Literally "the way," the term indicates how things develop naturally, nature moves along in its regular patterns, and living beings continuously grow and decline. Dao is the one power underlying all. The fundamental ground of being, it makes things what they are and causes the world to develop. Mysterious and ineffable, it cannot be known but only intuited in tranquil introspection. As the *Daode jing* says:

> Look at it and do not see it: we call it invisible.
> Listen to it and do not hear it: we call it inaudible.
> Touch it and do not feel it: we call it subtle. . . .
> Infinite and boundless, it cannot be named; . . .
> Vague and obscure,
> Meet it, yet you cannot see its head,
> Follow it, yet you cannot see its back. (ch. 14)

Beyond this, like *prakṛti,* Dao also manifests actively in the material, natural world and is clearly visible in rhythmic changes and patterned processes. On this, the phenomenal level, it is predictable in its developments and can be characterized as the give and take of various pairs of complementary opposites, as the natural ebb and flow of things as they rise and fall, come and go, grow and decline, emerge and die (Kohn 2005, 10). Like practitioners of Yoga, Daoists and Daoyin practitioners locate the human body-mind in the underlying cosmic continuum, as it is both the root of creation and manifest in the phenomenal world. Practitioners of either system strive to increase awareness of the fundamental structure and organization of reality, deepening their understanding of the fluid nature of the phenomenal world and encouraging the development of intuitive faculties that allow a greater appreciation of the underlying ground.

There is, therefore, a basic commonality in the elementary worldview underlying Yoga and Daoyin. However, there are also major differences. Unlike in Daoism, the Yogic ground of *prakṛti* is equipped with particular characteristics, qualities, or aspects known as *guṇas,* which are the ultimate building blocks of all material and mental phenomena. These are *sattva,* intelligence or luminosity that can reveal the ultimate but may also lead to attachment to knowledge and happiness; *rajas,* motor energy, passion, and activity which bind people to wealth and pleasures; and *tamas,* static inertia or ignorance that creates sloth, laziness, and delusion (Eliade 1969, 31; Feuerstein 1980, 33; Worthington 1982, 51).

These three condition psychological and physical life, and each manifest in five further aspects of reality. That is to say, *sattva,* the intelligent quality of *prakṛti,* appears in the five senses of perception, i.e., hearing, seeing, touching, smelling, and tasting. The motor energy or *rajas* of the primordial ground is activated in the five organs of action, i.e., hands, feet, speech, excretion, and reproduction. And the inert quality of *tamas* appears in the five *tanmātras* or birth states of the five elements—ether, gas, light, liquids, and solids—which join together to create the material world (Mishra 1987, xxv; Feuerstein 1980, 30).

In Daoism, on the contrary, Dao manifests in the two complementary forces yin and yang 陰陽 which originally described geographical features and were first used to indicate the shady and sunny sides of a hill. From there they acquired a series of associations: dark and bright, heavy and light, weak and strong, below and above, earth and heaven, minister and ruler, female and male, and so on. In concrete application, moreover, they came to indicate different kinds of action:

yang	active	birth	impulse	move	change	expand
yin	structive	completion	response	rest	nurture	contract

In addition, the ongoing flux and interchange of yin and yang was understood to occur in a series of five phases, which were symbolized by five materials or concrete entities:

minor yang	major yang	yin-yang	minor yin	major yin
wood	fire	earth	metal	water

These five energetic phases and their material symbols were then associated with a variety of entities in the concrete world, creating a complex system of correspondences. They were linked with colors, directions, seasons, musical tones, and with various functions in the human body, such as energy-storing (yin) organs, digestive (yang) organs, senses, emotions, and flavors. The basic chart at the root of Chinese and Daoist cosmology is as follows:

yin/yang	phase	direct.	color	season	organ1	organ2	emotion	sense
lesser yang	wood	east	green	spring	liver	gall	anger	eyes
greater yang	fire	south	red	summer	heart	sm. int.	exc. joy	tongue
yin-yang	earth	center	yellow		spleen	stomach	worry	lips
lesser yin	metal	west	white	fall	lungs	lg.int.	sadness	nose
greater yin	water	north	black	winter	kidneys	bladder	fear	ears

Daoyin practice, as much as other forms of Daoist body cultivation, accordingly aims to create perfect harmony among these various forces and patterns, which guarantees health and long life. Going beyond this harmony, adepts also hope to enter a deeper awareness of and oneness with the Dao at the center of creation, finding perfection through resting in and flowing along with the root of all being.

Yogic practice, in a quite different mode, does not work toward harmony with the *guṇas* and their various aspects, but sees them as obstacles that have to be overcome in order to reach the highest goal. The highest goal, moreover, is not the attainment of *prakṛti* in its aspect as the creative root of the world, but to go beyond *prakṛti* altogether to a level that is unique to the Indian system and has no matching counterpart in China. This level is described variously as *puruṣa, ātman, brahman,* and *īśvara.*

Puruṣa is best known from *Ṛgveda* hymns as the cosmic giant whose body is dismembered to create the world, a story that appears in Chinese folklore as the myth of Pangu 盤古 but which has little impact on Daoist practice (see Lincoln 1975; Mair 2004, 91).[1] *Puruṣa* is the original man, the cosmic creator, the cause of all material being and existence of the universe, the source of the source, the power behind even the underlying ground (Feuerstein 1980, 16). A representation of the sheer awareness that transcends even pure consciousness, *puruṣa* is the authentic, ultimate being of humanity, the far-off and detached seer of all ongoing psychic and physical processes, the perfect knowledge of all, the ultimate mirror of reality that is utterly apart, completely other, unmoving, unthinking, unfeeling, and unintending (Feuerstein 1980, 19-20).

In this latter sense, the notion of *puruṣa* in the *Ṛgveda* is very similar to the concept of *ātman* in the *Upanishads*, a collection of over a hundred philosophical writings based on the hermit tradition that dates from around 600 B.C.E. and are considered among the most sacred scriptures of Hinduism (see Kinsley 1989). Their key concept of *ātman*, which is used interchangeably with *puruṣa* in yogic texts, indicates the soul or true self, a transcendent autonomous principle that is unique, universal, fundamentally real, solidly substantial, and eternally free. Originally referring to the extended self, i.e., the social and individual personality, *ātman* first included the physical body as much as social status, family, and self-image. In the *Upanishads*, however, it came to be seen on a more sophisticated meditative level as the core of the individual's inner being, the divine moment within. Ultimately indestructible, *ātman* exists from the beginning of time and to the end of all eons. However often reincarnated and immersed in *prakṛti*, it remains forever free from evil, grief, hunger, thirst, old age, and death.

Ātman is so far beyond the senses and the intellect that it cannot be described, but one can pursue a state of consciousness that allows a glimpse. The *Mandukya Upanishad* distinguishes four kinds of consciousness—waking, dreaming, deep sleep, and meditative trance—noting that only the latter is a state that is awake yet completely free

---

[1] The *Ṛgveda* is the oldest and most important of the Four Vedas, which go back to about 3000-2000 B.C.E., and served as the key sacrificial hymn-books of Indo-Aryan culture, a parallel culture to the ancient Indus Valley civilization. Without spelling out philosophical doctrines, the texts imply notions of self-effacement and purity. See Kinsley 1989; Feuerstein 1998a.

from bodily concerns (Worthington 1982, 25). Like the wind, the clouds, lightning, and thunder, this state is present but does not rely on a tangible body that is subject to the limitations of the *guṇas*. Only in meditative trance can one experience the deepest inner nucleus of one's being, the ultimate true self or *ātman*. Deeply serene, one can allow the true self to shine forth in bright radiance (see Cope 2000). As the *Brihadaranyaka Upanishad* says:

> The true nature of the ultimate self is to be free from fear, free from desire and evil. As lovers in deep embrace forget everything, and only feel peace all around, so man where he embraces his true self feels peace all around. In that state there is neither father nor mother, there are no gods, no worlds, no good, and no evil. He neither sees, hears, tastes, smells, knows, nor touches. Yet he can see, for sight and he are one; he can hear, for sound and he are one. . . . (Worthington 1982, 16)

Ātman, moreover, is to be realized as ultimately one with *brahman*, the universal cosmic energy that is at the root beyond creation, is completely separate and different from all that exists materially, and is perceptible with the senses. *Brahman* is described as being in the world like salt is in water or like clay is in statues (Worthington 1982, 18), but in its original form it is utterly beyond description. It is

> not coarse, not fine, not short, not long, not glowing like fire, not adhesive like water, not bright, not dark, not airy, not spacious, not sticky, not tangible. It cannot be seen, nor heard, not smelled nor tasted. It is without voice and wind, without energy and breath, without measure, without number, without inside, without outside. (Worthington 1982, 25)

Brahman is the cosmic counterpart, the larger version of *ātman*, and a key doctrine of the ancient Indian thought that both are originally one. The goal of Yoga, then, as much as of other Indian ascetic practices and philosophies, is to fully realize that one's innermost, original, and perfect self is the same as the innermost, original, and perfect power of the universe. This is classically expressed in the phrase "Tat twam asi!" (Thou art that!)

The practice of Yoga accordingly is to move through different layers of the apparent self as created by and perceptible through *prakṛti* to come to the ultimate true self which is *puruṣa*, the original man, *ātman*, the innermost soul, and *brahman*, the underlying power of the universe. The key layers of the apparent self are the five so-called sheaths (*kośa*). They are: the physical body that is nourished by food;

the etheric body that exists through vital energy or *prāṇa*; the astral body made up from thoughts and intentions; the causal body consisting of pure intellect and knowledge; and the ultimate bliss body, true self, or *ātman* (Cope 2000, 68; Worthington 1982, 23; Mishra 1987, 49).

Yogic practice aims to reach oneness with *brahman*, to return to the purity of the original soul, and to recover the true self. Firm, fixed, permanent, and eternal, this true self is thus the person's ultimate identity. Originally one with the deepest transcendent ground of all, human beings have forgotten this identity through their karmic involvement with the world and the sensory experience of *prakṛti*. Through Yoga they can recover the innate stability, wholeness, and permanence of the cosmos within and return to the essential substance of their being.

To do so, in additional to regular practice, they also have to have strong devotion to *īśvara*, the lord, a personalized form of *brahman* who can extend grace and support to the practitioner. Omnipresent and omnitemporal, he remains pure, distant, and incomprehensible, yet in the yogic system "the grace of the deity is a necessary precondition for the recompense of ascetic exertion" (Feuerstein 1980, 4). *Īśvara* is innate cosmic enlightenment, coessential with the innermost self, the personified power that creates, upholds, and withdraws. Yoga is, therefore, essentially theistic (Eliade 1969, 16). Grace and devotion are key factors for success, and *īśvara praṇidhāna*, "refuge in the lord," is one of the five *niyamas*, the mental attitudes to be cultivated as the very foundation of the practice, which also include purity, contentment, austerity, and self-study.

With this strong otherworldly and theistic orientation, Yoga in its philosophical foundations is clearly different from the underlying vision of Daoyin. The Daoist universe is complex in its own way, similarly presupposes several layers of existence, and acknowledges the pervasive presence of an underlying ground; but it does not propose the substantial, eternal presence of something totally other. Daoist practice, as a result, remains within the realm of energetic refinement and transformation. Practitioners transmute into pure spirit, a subtle form of energy that flows at high velocity and allows easy transformations, celestial consciousness, and supernatural powers, but that is not utterly different from the world or a permanent, firm, unchanging entity of a transcendent nature.

The emphasis on the stability and permanence of the true self and the ultimate state in Yoga thus stand in radical contrast to the refinement into subtler and faster energetic flows in Daoyin. This difference, moreover, is also expressed in the execution of postures—a strong focus on stability and holding in Yoga as opposed to a sense of flow and easy movement in Daoyin—and in the role of the mind, which is the key subject of transformation in Yoga and an adjunct to transformation in Daoyin. Beyond that, the difference also manifests in the historical and social development of the two traditions.

History and Society

The historical origins of the two systems could not be more different. Yoga comes from the ancient Indian hermit tradition which "rejected the world as it is and devalued life as ephemeral, anguished, and ultimately illusory" (Eliade 1969, 18). Daoyin, on the other hand, arose as part of Han-dynasty medicine which encouraged people to relish the world in all its aspects, to find greater health, and to enjoy their physical and social pleasures. Both traditions have, in the course of their history, moved into the other realm—Yoga becoming a vehicle for health and Daoyin being integrated into the quest for immortality—but their origins and social bases remain far apart.

The earliest document on Yoga is the *Yogasūtras* of Patañjali, who may or may not be identical with a well-known Sanskrit grammarian who lived around 300 B.C.E. The date of both author and text is unclear, and some scholars have placed them as late as the third century C.E., but all agree that the text is later than the *Upanishads* and early Buddhism and probably came after the *Bhagavad Gita* (Worthington 1982, 55). The text divides into four main sections on Yogic Ecstasy, Discipline, Miraculous Powers, and Isolation (Eliade 1969, 12), and consists of 196 *sūtras* or short half-sentences that are more mnemonic aids than clarifying explanations (Taimni 1975, viii). It is largely philosophical in nature and inherits key doctrines from the *Vedas* and *Upanishads*.

For example, an important *sūtra* that is often cited among yogis today appears right in the beginning: "Yoga is the cessation of the modifications of the mind" or the "abolition of all states of consciousness" (I.2). I. K. Taimni writes a four-page explanation on this short phrase, dwelling on every word and reaching the conclusion that its intended meaning refers to the overcoming, through yogic practice, of the various states and delusions of the mind that are conditioned by the *guṇas* and thus opening the way to the appreciation and realization of *ātman* (1975, 6-10). Mircea Eliade sees the phrase as describing the gradual overcoming and elimination of all errors, delusions, and dreams, then of all normal psychological experiences, and finally even of all parapsychological powers to the point of complete cessation (1969, 51). Confirming this, the text moves on to explain the various trance states in the depth of meditative absorption and the need to overcome the *guṇas* and identify fully with *puruṣa*. As this example shows, the text is brief in phrasing and often obscure. Thus Georg Feuerstein says: "Their extreme brevity and conciseness renders the *sūtras* almost unintelligible to the uninitiated" while at the same time guaranteeing "the great degree of flexibility witnessed in the diverse traditions" of Yoga (1979, 21).

In contrast to this rather obscure and philosophical writing, the earliest works on Daoyin are immensely practical in nature and can be precisely dated. Found among manuscripts unearthed from southern China, they include the silk manuscript *Daoyin tu* 導引圖 (Exercise Chart) and the bamboo tablets of the *Yinshu* 引書 (Stretch Book).

The *Daoyin tu* was found at Mawangdui, in the tomb of the Marchioness of Dai, the wife of a local lord who died in 168 B.C.E. The text consists of forty-four color illustrations of human figures performing

therapeutic exercises that are explained in brief captions (see Fig. 1). The figures are of different sex and age, variously clothed or bare-chested, and shown in different postures (mostly standing) from a variety of angles. In many cases, they have one arm reaching up while the other stretches down, one arm moving forward while the other extends back, possibly indicating rhythmical movement.

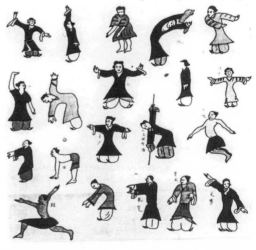

Fig. 1: The Mawangdui "Exercise Chart."

There is some variety among them. Two figures are in a forward bend, one with head lowered, the other with head raised. Another is bending slightly forward with a rounded back and hands hanging down toward the knees. Yet another has one arm on the ground and the other extended upward in a windmill-like pose (Harper 1998, 132). The captions are often illegible, but among them are the well-known "bear amble" and "bird stretch," showing a figure walking in a stately fashion with arms swinging and one bending forward with hands on the floor and head raised, respectively.

The lack of written explanations is somewhat alleviated by the *Yinshu*, which consists entirely of text. It was found in a manuscript at Zhangjiashan 張家山, also in Hunan, in a tomb that was closed in 186 B.C.E. The text divides into three parts: a general introduction on seasonal health regimens; a series of about a hundred exercises, divided into three sections; and a conclusion on the etiology of disease and ways of prevention (see Fig. 2).

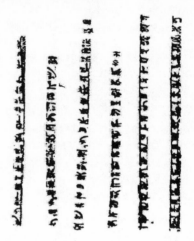

Fig.2: The "Stretch Book".

The first part on seasonal health regimens discusses hygiene, diet, sleep, and movement as well as adequate times for sexual intercourse. It is ascribed to Pengzu 彭祖, a famous immortal of antiquity, said to have lived over 800 years. It says, for instance:

> Spring days. After rising in the morning, pass water, wash and rinse, clean and click the teeth. Loosen the hair, stroll to the lower end of the hall to meet the purest of dew and receive the essence of Heaven, and drink one cup of water. These are the means to increase accord. Enter the chamber [for sex] between evening until greater midnight [1 a.m.]. More would harm the *qi*. (Harper 1998, 110-11; Engelhardt 2001, 215)

This places the practice firmly in the home of a wealthy aristocrat with leisure to pursue long life and well-being and the inclination to perform proper hygiene and develop bodily awareness. It also assumes that the practitioner lives in society and has a wife or concubine for bedroom activities. The scene could not be farther removed from the kind of hermit setting that lies at the foundation of Yoga.

Following a general outline of daily routines, the middle part of the *Yinshu* provides concrete practice instructions, describing and naming specific moves. For example:

> "Bend and Gaze" is: interlace the fingers at the back and bend forward, then turn the head to look at your heels (#12).

> "Dragon Flourish" is: step one leg forward with bent knee while stretching the other leg back, then interlace the fingers, place them on the knee, and look up (#19).

> "Pointing Backward" is: interlace the fingers, raise them overhead and bend back as far as possible (#29).[2]

Following forty exercises of this type, the text focuses on the medical use of the practices. It often repeats instructions outlined earlier and in some cases prescribes a combination of them. For example, a variation of lunges such as "Dragon Flourish" is the following, which can be described as a walking lunge:

> To relieve tense muscles: Stand with legs hip-width apart and hold both thighs. Then bend the left leg while stretching the right thigh back, reaching the knee to the floor. Once done, [change legs and] bend the right leg while stretching the left leg back and reaching that knee to the floor. Repeat three times (#46).

Another variant of the lunges is recommended to relieve *qi* disruptions in the muscles and intestines. Lunging with the left foot forward and the right leg back, one goes into a twist by bending the right arm at the elbow and looking back over the left shoulder. After three repetitions on both sides, one is to maintain the lunge position while raising one arm at a time and then both arms up as far as one can (each three times), bending the back and opening the torso (#68). The idea seems to be that by stretching arms and legs one can open blockages in the extremities while the twisting of the abdominal area aids the intestines.

Exercises like these in the medical section of the text also include breathing techniques, notably exhalations with *chui*, *xu*, and *hu* (three forms of the six breaths) to strengthen the body and to harmonize *qi*-flow, as well as exercises in other than standing positions, such as seated, kneeling, or lying down. For example, to alleviate

---

[2] These translations are based on the original text. It is published with modern characters and some punctuation in Wenwu 1990; Ikai 2004.

lower back pain, one should lie on one's back and rock the painful area back and forth 300 times—if possible with knees bent into the chest. After this, one should lift the legs up straight to ninety degrees, point the toes, and—with hands holding on to the mat—vigorously lift and lower the buttocks three times (#55).

An example of a kneeling practice is the following:

> To relieve thigh pain. Kneel upright, stretch the left leg for- ward while rotating the right shoulder down to bring them together with some vigor. Then stretch the right leg forward while rotating the left shoulder down to bring them together. Repeat ten times. (#50)

Following this detailed outline of concrete exercises, the *Yinshu* con- cludes its third part with a list of twenty-four brief mnemonic state- ments. After this, it places the practice into a larger social and cul- tural context. It notes that the most important factors in causing dis- eases are climatic excesses:

> People get sick because of heat, dampness, wind, cold, rain, or dew as well as because of [a dysfunction] in opening and closing the pores, a disharmony in eating and drinking, and the inability to adapt their rising and resting to the changes in cold and heat. (Engelhardt 2001, 216)

This harks back to the seasonal regimen in the beginning of the text, restating the importance of climatic and temporal awareness in the way one treats the body. The proper way of treating the body, how- ever, as the text points out next, is accessible mainly to "noble people" of the upper classes, who fall ill because of uncontrolled emotions such as anger and joy (which overload yin and yang *qi*). "Base peo- ple," whose conditions tend to be caused by excessive labor, hunger, and thirst, on the contrary, have no opportunity to learn the neces- sary breathing exercises and therefore contract numerous diseases and die early.

This, as much as the fact that the manuscripts were found in tombs of local rulers, makes it clear that Daoyin practice in Han China was very much the domain of the aristocracy and upper classes and aimed predominantly at alleviating diseases and physical discomforts, pro- viding greater enjoyment of daily luxuries and faster recovrery after raucous parties (Engelhardt 2000, 88; 2001, 217; also Harper 1995, 381). Also, the very existence of the texts with their detailed instruc- tions shows that the practices were public knowledge and accessible to anyone with enough interest and financial means to obtain them.

Historical records show that medical and philosophical materials were often collected by aristocrats. Some searched out already written works and had them transcribed; others invited knowledgeable people to their estate and had them dictate their philosophical sayings and medical recipes to an experienced scribe. While knowledge was transmitted orally in a three-year apprenticeship from father to son in professional medical families or from master to disciple among itinerant practitioners and within philosophical schools, the dominant tendency was to offer this knowledge to society at large, and there was little concern for the establishment of close-knit hierarchies or esoteric lineages (Harper 1998, 61).

The situation in Indian Yoga is much different. As the *Yogasūtras* reflect, the masters' knowledge, however practical, was closely guarded and formulated in obscure philosophical phrases. Disciples had to commit fully to their teacher, and together with faith in the grace of *īśvara* had to have total trust in and obedience to the guru who, as representative of the ultimate, possessed powers far beyond ordinary knowledge (see Arya 1981; Hewitt 1977). Also, since the goal of Yoga was the attainment of complete cessation of mentation and the realization of the transcendent true self, it could not be undertaken within society—let alone be used for the enhancement of ordinary pleasures. The only way to freedom and beatitude in Yoga, as Mircea Eliade points out, was to withdraw from the world, detach from wealth and ambition, and live in radical self-isolation (1969, 21).

Socially, therefore, Yoga took place in a completely different context than Daoyin. Yogic practitioners were not aristocrats trying to stay healthy and have more fun, but radical ascetics who denied themselves even the most basic human comforts. The ascetic hermit (*sadhu*) would give up all products of culture and live in the wilderness, not even "stepping on ploughed land," the symbol of human domination over nature (Olivelle 1990, 133). He—very few if any female ascetics are mentioned from the early stages (Ghurye 1964, 40)—would eat only uncultivated foods, such as fruits, berries, roots, and herbs; wear bark, leaves, and animal skins; leave his hair unkempt and his nails growing; and imitate animals in his behavior—notably deer, cows, pigeons, fish, snakes, and dogs. Returning to a state of primal origin, before the plow and social hierarchies, he would find paradise for himself in utter independence from society (Olivelle 1990, 134-35). Thus he could attain the freedom of mind and body necessary for ultimate release.

Typically such ascetics undertook a variety of practices, which are still familiar among the yogis of today.

> There are those who squatted on their heels, others who lay on beds of thorns, ashes or grass, others who rested on a pestle. . . . One was avowedly following the vow of exposing himself to the elements, especially to the sun and the rain. Another with the help of a long staff was carrying out the austerity of standing on one leg. (Ghurye 1964, 39-40)

This contrasts vividly with the description of the ideals of Daoyin from a fourth-century text, which through its very warning of the enticements of sensuality and beauty shows just how much its practitioners were exposed to them. It says,

> The method of nourishing longevity consists mainly in not doing harm to oneself. Keep warm in winter and cool in summer, and never lose your harmony with the four seasons—that is how you can align yourself with the body. Do not allow sensuous beauty, provocative postures, easy leisure, and enticing entertainments to incite yearnings and desires—that is how you come to pervade the spirit. (Stein 1999, 169)

Rather than subject themselves to extremes, practitioners of Daoyin matched the changes of nature, creating harmony in the body and in society instead of leaving the family and restructuring the body to the point of complete cessation. The physical and breathing exercises of the two systems, however apparently similar, in their original setting thus served completely different purposes, were executed in completely different social milieus, and found expression in completely different kinds of documents.

Healing and Transcendence

As history moved along, this original contrast between the two traditions began to dissolve to a certain degree. Daoyin became part of the Daoist enterprise of the attainment of immortality and Yoga, as we know all too well from its popularity today, turned into a major method for health and well-being. How and when did this change occur?

In the case of Daoyin, it had to do with the arising of various organized Daoist groups that adopted some self-cultivation methods practiced by Chinese hermits (see Kohn 2001). Most prominent among them was the school of Highest Clarity (Shangqing 上清), which arose in the 360s, when two brothers of the aristocratic Xu family hired the medium Yang Xi 楊羲 (330–386) to establish contact with Xu Mi's 許 謐 wife who had died in 362 to find out about her fate in the other-world. She appeared to tell them about her status and explained the overall organization of the heavens. She also introduced the medium to various other spirit figures who revealed methods of personal transformation, meditations, visualizations, and alchemical concoctions; gave thorough instructions on how to transmit the texts and their methods; and provided prophecies about the golden age to come (see Strickmann 1981).

The Xu brothers wrote down everything Yang Xi transmitted, however disparate it may have seemed, and created a basic collection of sacred texts. They shared their new revelations with their immediate neighbors and relatives, thus establishing the first generation of Highest Clarity followers (Robinet 1984, 1:108). They developed a spiritual practice that also included a daily routine of stretches, breathing, and self-massages in combination with the use of talismans and incantations—all to purify their bodies and to enhance their vigor for the great endeavor of becoming immortal.

How Daoyin functioned in the daily practice of these would-be immortals is described in the *Baoshen jing* 寶神經 (Scripture on Treasuring the Spirit, DZ 1319; see Robinet 1984, 2:359-62). The text says:

> When you get up in the morning, always calm your breath and sit up straight, then interlace the fingers and massage the nape of your neck. Next, lift the face and look up, press the hands against the neck while moving the head back. Do this three or four times, then stop.[3]

> This causes essence to be in harmony and the blood to flow well. It prevents wind or wayward *qi* from entering the body. Over a long time it will keep you free from disease and death.

> Next, bend and stretch; extend the hands to the four extremes [up, down, right, left]; bend backward and stretch

---

[3] The same exercise is still part of the Daoyin repertoire today. It appears under the name "Immortal Imitating Tall Pine Standing Firmly in the Wind" in Ni Hua-ching's regimen (1989, 60). Here the posture proposed is to sit cross-legged.

out the sides; and shake out the hundred joints. Do each of these three times. (6a)

These and similar morning practices were further accompanied by incantations that implored the deities and perfected to support the practitioner and enhanced their visions of divine ascension. An example is:

My spirit and material souls receiving purity,
My five spirits [of the inner organs] are restful and at peace.
I return in a flying carriage to visit [the heaven of] Jade Clarity,
Ascend to Great Nonbeing and journey with the sun.
Becoming a perfected, I merge in mystery with emperors and lords. (2b)

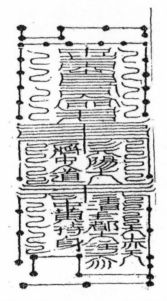

The practice also involved the use of talismans, written in red ink on yellow paper in imitation of the sacred writings of the otherworld. Adepts used them either by placing them on themselves or by burning them and drinking the ashes (*Baoshen jing* 16b) (see Fig. 3).

The morning practices of Daoyin in Highest Clarity served several goals: dispersal of obstructive and demonic forces, self-purification in the face of the divine, clarity of vision and keenness of hearing to open otherworldly perception, extension of life expectancy to have more practice time, and preparation for ascension through visualizations of gods and heavens (see Robinet 1993).

Fig. 3: A talisman used in Highest Clarity practice.

Variations of the practice include:

- bends and stretches known from the medical manuscripts as well as deep breathing to release stale *qi* and absorb new energy;

- self-massages of the face, eyes, and ears;

- saliva swallowings to harmonize *qi* in the body and calm the viscera;

- visualizations of the inner organs with the body gods.

In this religious Daoist context, therefore, the practice of Daoyin was transformed into an aspect of spiritual purification, including but not limited to the maintenance of health and extension of life. Although the setting was still aristocratic and mundane, it has come much closer to Yoga, leading to extensive explorations of the unseen world and deep absorptive trance states.[4]

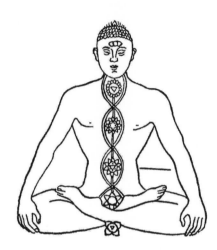

Yoga, on the other hand, moved in the opposite direction, leading to a greater emphasis on health benefits and a wider spread among people within society. Two movements in particular took the tradition into a more secular environment and transformed it into a popular form of self-therapy. The first is known as Laya Yoga. It arose toward the end of the first millennium C.E. as part of the tantric adoption of Yoga and focused on utilizing the energy that arises in the body after prolonged meditation.

Fig. 4: The Seven Chakras in the body.

This energy, called *kundalini*, was thought to lie dormant at the base of the spine. If awakened properly, it would begin to move from here, rising up along the spine through three major *nadis* or energy channels. Along the way it would open the seven *chakras* or energy centers until it reached the top of the head where it would unify with cosmic consciousness and exit the body (see Fig. 4). By activating *kundalini*, the belief was, people could bring their energetic system

---

[4] This more spiritual form of Daoyin practice has persisted in the Daoist tradition, leading to the integration of gymnastic exercises into later forms of Daoist meditation and immortality practice, including the complex system of inner alchemy—the creation of an elixir and immortal embryo within the body—which still is the dominant form of Daoist spiritual practice today (see Berk 1986; Despeux 1988). On the other hand, it has also recovered its medical origins in the practice of Qigong, which since the 1950s has adopted Daoist techniques into a health regimen for the masses and spread successfully not only throughout China but also in East Asia and the West (see Kohn forthcoming).

into balance and reach greater health, endurance, and well-being (Worthington 1982, 100-02).

The seven chakras, moreover, were associated with various colors, geometric forms or *yantras*, deities, and personality types. They are:[5]

Name	Location	Color	Yantra	Personality	Deity
Root	perineum	red	square	survival	Brahma
Sacral	abdomen	orange	semi-circle	creativity	Vishnu
Central	solar plexus	yellow	triangle	ego/confidence	Rudra
Heart	chest/thyroid	pink	star	love/compassion	Isha
Throat	throat/pineal	blue	triangle	logic/thought	Shiva
Brow	third eye	violet	circle	intuition	
Crown	top of head	gold	triangle	spirituality	

Activating the *chakras* through a mixture of physical practices, breathing exercises, and meditations, practitioners hoped to find perfect balance in their energetic system to create health, vigor, and long life. As history moved on, however, the practice was once more reintegrated with the higher spiritual goals of Patañjali's *Yogasūtras* and practitioners came to aspire to advanced stages of evolution, reaching out to complete transcendence and the true self. Even the awakening of the *kundalini* eventually came to be described as a mystical, supernatural experience. As the modern mystic Krishna Gopi records:

> I experienced a rocking sensation and then felt myself slipping out of my body, entirely enveloped in a halo of light. I felt the point of consciousness that was myself growing wider, surrounded by waves of light. I was not all consciousness, without any outline, without any idea of a corporeal appendage, without any feeling or sensation coming from the senses, immersed in a sea of light. (1977, 143)

Therefore, while Laya Yoga may have begun as a secularized form of energy transformation, it eventually recovered the spiritual aspects of classical Yoga and became an important part of the tantric tradition (see Feuerstein 1998a).

This is not quite the case in the other therapy form of Yoga, known as Hatha Yoga and named after a combination of *ha*, the sun, and *tha*, the moon, meant to indicate the joining and harmonizing of the two basic forms of energy in the body (Yasudian and Haich 1965, 20).

Hatha Yoga goes back to a group known as Nath yogis who flourished in northern India from the tenth century onward. Founded by Goruk-

---

[5] See Wood 1962, 153-55; Worthington 1982, 104-06; Yasudian and Haich 1965, 93-95

sanatha, this group placed great emphasis on physical fitness, developed various forms of martial arts, and engaged in psychic experiments. Rather than remain aloof from society, they made attempts at reform, treating women and outcasts as equals and trying to unite Hindus and Buddhists. Their efforts were not greatly appreciated by the ruling classes, and they were soon relegated to a lower caste. Still, the legendary Gurkha fighters are said to be their heirs, and their transformation of Yoga into an art of practical living has had a profound impact on the tradition (Worthington 1982, 129).

The main document of the Nath yogis is the *Hathayoga pradīpikā* (Light on Hatha Yoga), which was compiled in the fifteenth century on the basis of the notes and instructions of earlier masters by Svatmarama Swami, also known as Divatma Ram. Arranged in five sections on Initial Practices, Stepping up Energy, Overcoming Limitations, Manifesting Self, and Corrective Treatments, it is written like the *Yogasūtras* in a series of short instructions that need further personal instruction (Worthington 1982, 129).

Unlike the *Yogasūtras* and more like the early Daoyin manuscripts, however, the *Hathayoga pradīpikā* is eminently practical and quite concrete. It warns against excesses that will hinder the practice, including overeating, exertion, useless talk, extreme abstinence, public company, and unsteadiness of mind. Instead it encourages persistence, knowledge, courage, and determination (Worthington 1982, 130). It follows the eight limbs of the *Yogasūtras* but places a stronger emphasis on moral discipline and the physical practices than on deep absorptions and meditative trances. It supports the five *yamas* or restraints—against killing, stealing, lying, sexual misconduct, and attachments—and the five *niyamas* or proper mental attitudes: purity, contentment, austerity, self-study, and refuge in the lord (Iyengar 1976, 31-40). Continuing along the eight limbs, the text then provides detailed instructions on the performance of fifteen key postures or *āsanas* and moves on to a discussion of breath control or *pranayāma* (Eliade 1969, 65).

Hatha Yoga has become dominant in the practice of Yoga today and for many people means the creation of perfect health, defined as the state of natural equilibrium of all energies and the free flow of *prāna*, the inner life force that smoothes out irregularities and preserves health, the power of gravity, attraction, repulsion, electricity, and radioactivity (Yasudian and Haich 1965, 30, 53).

Prana is more concrete and more tangible than *kundalini*; present in everyone and everything, it does not need to be awakened. Very much like *qi*, it is omnipresent, flows through energy channels in the body, and is activated through conscious breathing and controlled physical movements. People tend to neglect and waste their *prāna*, straining it through exhausting labor, excessive sexuality, and draining mental work—items that Daoists would heartily endorse. Hatha Yoga, like Daoyin, accordingly teaches to use and store vital energy to the maximum, thereby enhancing health and extending long life (Yasudian and Haich 1965, 36, 31).

The proper use of *prana* ultimately leads to the complete control over the body and mind, the ability to counteract various outside influences through internal energy work and to overcome and eventually eliminate all sorts of harmful emotions, such as rage, fear, grief, sorrow, fright, jealousy, despondency, and pessimism (Yasudian and Haich 1965, 37). While this may again sound very much like the program of Daoyin or even Qigong, the ultimate goal of Hatha Yoga is formulated once more in the classical vision as the ultimate transformation of consciousness. As B. K. S. Iyengar notes:

> Yoga is the method by which the restless mind is calmed and the energy directed into constructive channels. . . . The mind, when controlled, provides a reservoir of peace and generates abundant energy for human uplift. . . .
>
> [Eventually] the seer, the sight, and the seen have no separate existence from each other. It is like a great musician becoming one with his instrument and the music that comes from it. Then the yogi stands in his own nature and realizes his true self, the part of the Supreme Soul within himself. (1976, 20, 22)

Divergent Techniques

Taking all this information together, we can now begin to answer the questions posed in the beginning. Are Yoga and Daoyin essentially the same but formulated differently? Or are they two separate traditions that have very little in common? It should be clear by now that in their original social setting, cosmological speculation, and textual formulation they are very different indeed, although they share some basic notions about the nature of existence and propose similar physical practices. In the course of history, on the other hand, they have come a bit closer to each other, Daoyin being used in a more spiritual context and Yoga transforming into popular therapy. This shift has also led to a certain change in key concepts, Laya and Hatha Yoga emphasizing notions of internal vital energy that are very much like *qi*, and Highest Clarity and later Daoists engaging in deep trance states with the hope to reach otherworldly dimensions.

To conclude this discussion, I would now like to take a closer look at the actual practices and their commonalities and differences. First, quite obviously, both Yoga and Daoyin support a moderate and simple lifestyle, a nutritious and natural diet, freedom from strong emotions, and clarity in daily living. They have a basic moral code, formulated as the *yamas* and *niyamas* in Yoga and apparent in Daoism in various sets of precepts for lay followers, priests, and monastics (see Kohn 2004).

Both also prescribe a fairly straightforward exercise regimen that, combined with deep, abdominal and chest-expanding breathing, can be executed in all different positions of the body. Exercises include bends and stretches, most commonly forward bends, backbends, lunges, and twists, as well as some weight-bearing practices, such as pull-ups and push-ups. Many of these basic exercises are part and parcel of any workout routine and will be familiar to athletes and gym-users everywhere. They have been proven effective for health over many centuries and in all different cultures, just as a moderate life style and good moral foundation have been helpful all along.

So far, both systems do not contradict each other, nor are they different from other health enhancing methods, whether they emphasize the physical or the spiritual. Their effectiveness is not questioned, nor is their general applicability. Beyond this, however, things become more complicated. Both Yoga and Daoyin have more complex postures and sequences that are not at all alike in name or execution.[6]

Daoyin variously makes use of ropes and swings, which are not found in Yoga. Yoga, on the other hand, places a great emphasis on inversions and balancing poses which are strikingly absent in Daoyin. Also, with the exception of the meditation known as "Standing Like a Pine Tree," Daoyin tends to encourage movement, while Yoga demands holding—sometimes for periods of ten, twenty, or thirty minutes. This, of course, goes back to the ultimate goal in Yoga of reaching a level of complete inner stability that allows the awareness of the eternal true

---

[6] One exception is figure 44 on the *Daoyin tu*, shown with legs in lunge position and arms extended and named "Warrior Pointing," which is strikingly similar to the Yoga pose known as "Warrior II."

self, contrasted with the aim of Daoists to become one with the flow and to find perfect harmony by moving along with the patterns of Dao.

A similar set of differences also applies to the breathing practices associated with the two systems, *qifa* 氣法 in Daoyin and *pranayāma* in Yoga. Both encourage holding of the breath—called *biqi* 閉氣 in Daoyin and *kumbhaka* in Yoga—for the opening of energy channels. Both use a method of directed breathing to alleviate discomforts and distress, and both guide energy up the spinal column. Yet, in general Daoyin works with the systematic circulation of *qi* throughout the body, while Yoga focuses on the concentrated use of breath in the nostril, sinus, and throat areas.

For example, one form of Daoyin breathing is called "swallowing qi" (*yanqi* 咽氣). According to the *Huanzhen xiansheng fu neiqi juefa* 幻真先生服內氣訣法 (Master Huanzhen's Essential Method of Absorbing Internal *Qi*, DZ 828),[7] this involves lying flat on one's back with the head slightly raised and the hands curled into fists. In this position, adepts inhale through the nose, allow the breath to reach the mouth, mix it with saliva by moving the tongue and cheeks, and swallow it down, guiding the *qi* mentally to reach the stomach and spread from there into the various inner organs. To help the movement, practitioners massage the passageway of the breath by rubbing the chest and belly (2b-3b).

In an extension, they also "guide the *qi*" (*xingqi* 行氣) by first taking the swallowed saliva-breath mixture into the lower elixir field, then entering it into two small caverns at the back and imagining it moving up the body in two strands to enter the Niwan Center or upper elixir field in the head. From here they allow it to stream into all parts of the body, "through hair, face, head, neck, and shoulders into the hands and fingers; from the chest and the middle elixir field at the heart into the five inner organs and down along the legs to thighs, knees, calves, heels, and soles" (3b-4a). As they do so, all congestions of blood and blockages of *qi* are successfully dissolved, paving the way for the refinement of *qi* into subtler energetic forces.

A yet different variant is called "surrendering to qi" (weiqi 委氣), which is described as flowing mentally along with the qi in the body

---

[7] The text has a preface dated to the mid-Tang period. It also appears in the *Chifeng sui* 赤鳳髓 (Marrow of the Red Phoenix) of the late Ming. It is translated Despeux 1988, 65-81 and summarized in Kohn, forthcoming.

wherever it may go in a state of deep absorption, "where there is no spirit, no conscious awareness; deep and serene, the mind is one with the Great Void" (5b-6a). This in turn causes the body to become independent of nostril breathing as the *qi* will begin to flow through the pores of the skin. In an extension of this heightened power of *qi*, adepts can then spread it to other people in a form of laying-on of hands to create healing and greater harmony with the Dao.

In contrast to these breathing practices, Yoga followers use the breath to heighten awareness, to calm the mind, and to cleanse the air passages (see Loehr and Migdow 1986). To give a few examples, there is a popular form known as *ujjayi* breathing, often called the "ocean-sounding breath." It involves the tightening of the muscles at the back of the throat, allowing the air to flow slowly and making a soft, rasping noise, said to stimulate the endocrine and thyroid glands and increase mental alertness (Yasudian and Haich 1965, 120). A breath that calms the mind and balances energy channels is *nadi shodana*. Also called "alternate nostril breathing," it is done by alternately closing off one nostril with the fingers or thumb of the right hand. Encouraging long, calm inhalations and complete, deep exhalations, this is very soothing and aids the integration of the two brain hemispheres.

Another classic yogic breath is *bhastrikā*, which means "bellows." In this exercise, the breath is pushed in and out quickly and powerfully ten times, after which it is held in for 5-10 seconds. It is said to help with colds, destroy phlegm, relieve inflammation of the nose and throat, and over longer periods may cure asthma (Yasudian and Haich 1965, 122). The "skull-polishing" breath, finally, is called *kapalabhāti*. It cleanses and tones up the nasal passages, expels bacteria, and increases concentration. For this, practitioners breathe in deeply and then expel the breath in short bursts from the lungs through the nose while vigorously contracting the abdominal muscles and pushing the diaphragm upward. They continue for thirty to fifty repetitions, then exhale completely, hold the breath out while "securing the locks" by tightening the muscles in pelvis, belly, and throat, then inhale and hold the breath in (Yasudian 1965, 120-21).

This brief overview of the best known breathing practices in the two systems shows just how significantly different they are in both form and purpose. Daoists mix the breath with saliva and guide it internally to effect opening of *qi*-channels while Yogis work with strong, deep inhalations and exhalations to cleanse specific physical channels.

The difference is further enhanced by the vast variety in cleansing procedures in the two traditions. Daoists practice daily hygiene by washing the face, rinsing the mouth, and cleaning the teeth. They also expel stale *qi* upon waking in the morning. To do so, they close the eyes and curl their hands into fists. Lying down flat, they bend the arms and set the fists on the chest, while placing the feet on the mat to raise the knees. From here, they lift the back and buttocks, hold the breath in, and pound on the abdomen to make the stale *qi* in the belly flow back out through the mouth (*Huanzhen juefa* 1ab).

Yogis likewise wash and rinse and clean their teeth, but in addition they also gargle, rub the base of the tongue and cleanse it with butter, and clean the hole in the skull by massaging the third-eye area. They clean the interior of the chest by inserting a plantain stalk through the mouth into the esophagus and the nasal passages, hoping thereby to remove phlegm, mucus, and bile. They may also swallow a fine cloth about three inches wide, allowing it to reach the stomach, then pull it out again, or they might guide a thread through the nostrils into the mouth to open the sinuses. For intestinal sweepings, they push water in and out of the rectum or insert a stalk of turmeric into the colon (Wood 1971, 126-28). All these are methods quite unique to the Indian tradition that have no documented counterpart in China.

Conclusion

Given the enormous differences in historical origins, fundamental worldview, and applied techniques, it is safe to conclude that Yoga and Daoyin are indeed two radically different systems of body cultivation. This is despite the fact that there are certain basic similarities in body postures and energy circulation (Mair 2004, 88; 1990, 140-48); that there was rich cultural contact between Persia, India, and China already in the first millennium B.C.E.; that evidence shows the use of various technical Sanskrit terms in Chinese (Mair 2004, 92); and that Buddhist masters undoubtedly brought physical and breathing practices to China in addition to scriptures and meditations in the first few centuries C.E. (see Despeux 1989; Eliade 1958).

In spite of all this, examining the deeper levels of the two systems, it becomes clear that Yoga and Daoyin are completely at odds in the way they deal with the body:

- They see the body differently: Yogis strive to control and overcome its characteristics, while Daoyin followers hope to align with it and perfect its functioning.

- They use the body differently: Yogis change its natural patterns and ultimately aim to keep it quiet and stable for the unfolding of mental purity and a vision of the true self, while Daoyin practitioners enhance its natural functioning with the expectation of refining its energetic structure to greater levels of subtlety and thus reaching the perfection of the Dao.

- They heal the body differently: Yogis accept health as a byproduct and necessary condition for more advanced stages and—with the exception of Hatha practitioners—tend to scorn the pursuit of mere bodily well-being and successful functioning in society, while Daoyin masters—again with some exceptions in later Daoist circles—emphasize health, long life, and the experience of mundane pleasures and see them as a key motivation of the practice, more spiritual states being possible but not essential.

Both systems, when followed at a basic level, can help people find wellness in their bodies, peace in their minds, and balance in their lives. They both fulfill an important role in modern technological and hyperactive societies. However, when it comes to higher spiritual goals, their visions, organizational settings, and practices are vastly divergent.

Bibliography

Arya, Usharbudh. 1981. *Mantra and Meditation*. Honesdale, PA: Himalayan Institute.

Berk, William R. 1986. *Chinese Healing Arts: Internal Kung-Fu*. Burbank, Calif.: Unique Publications.

Cope, Stephen. 2000. *Yoga and the Quest for True Self*. New York: Bantam.

Despeux, Catherine. 1988. *La moélle du phénix rouge: Santé et longue vie dans la Chine du seiziéme siècle*. Paris: Editions Trédaniel.

_____. 1989. "Gymnastics: The Ancient Tradition." In *Taoist Meditation and Longevity Techniques*, edited by Livia Kohn, 223-61.

Ann Arbor: University of Michigan, Center for Chinese Studies Publications.

Eliade, Mircea. 1958. *Yoga: Immortality and Freedom*. New York: Pantheon Books.

_____.1969. *Patanjali and Yoga*. New York: Funk & Wagnalls.

Engelhardt, Ute. 2000. "Longevity Techniques and Chinese Medicine." In *Daoism Handbook*, edited by Livia Kohn, 74-108. Leiden: E. Brill.

_____. 2001. "*Daoyin tu* und *Yinshu*: Neue Erkenntnisse über die Übungen zur Lebenspflege in der frühen Han-Zeit." *Monumenta Serica* 49: 213-26.

Feuerstein, Georg. 1979. *The Yoga-Sūtra of Patañjali*. New Delhi: Arnold Heinemann.

_____. 1980. *The Philosophy of Classical Yoga*. New York: St. Martin's Press.

_____. 1998a. *Tantra: The Path of Ecstasy*. Boston: Shambhala.

_____. 1998b. *The Yoga Tradition: Its History, Literature, Philosophy and Practice*. Prescott, AZ: Hohm Press.

Ghurye, G. S. 1964. *Indian Sadhus*. Bombay: Popular Prakashan.

Gopi, Krishna. 1985. *Kundalini: The Evolutionary Energy in Man*. Boston: Shambhala.

Harper, Donald. 1998. *Early Chinese Medical Manuscripts: The Mawangdui Medical Manuscripts*. London: Wellcome Asian Medical Monographs.

Hewitt, James. 1977. *The Complete Yoga Book*. New York: Schocken Books.

Ikai Yoshio 豬飼祥夫. 2004. "Kōryō Chōkasan kanken Insho yakuchūkō" 江陵張家山漢簡引書釋註. Draft paper. Used by permission of the author.

Iyengar, B.K.S. 1976. *Light on Yoga*. New York: Schocken Books.

Kinsley, David R. 1989. *Hinduism: A Cultural Perspective*. Englewood Cliffs, NJ: Prentice Hall.

Kohn, Livia. 2001. *Daoism and Chinese Culture*. Cambridge: Three Pines Press.

_____. 2004. *Cosmos and Community: The Ethical Dimension of Daoism*. Cambridge, Mass.: Three Pines Press.

_____. 2005. *Health and Long Life: The Chinese Way*. In cooperation with Stephen Jackowicz. Cambridge, Mass.: Three Pines Press.

_____. forthcoming. *Chinese Healing Exercises*. Magdalena, NM: Three Pines Press.

Lincoln, Bruce. 1975. "The Indo-European Myth of Creation." *History of Religions* 15: 121-45.

Loehr, James E., and Jeffrey A. Migdow. 1986. *Breathe In, Breathe Out: Inhale Energy and Exhale Stress by Guiding and Controlling Your Breathing*. Alexandria, VA: Time Life Books.

Mair, Victor. 1990. *Tao Te Ching: The Classic Book of Integrity and the Way*. New York: Bantam.

_____. 2004. "The Beginnings of Sino-Indian Cultural Contact." *Journal of Asian History* 38.2: 81-96.

Mishra, Rammurti S. 1987. *Fundamentals of Yoga: A Handbook of Theory, Practice, and Application*. New York: Harmony Books.

Ni, Hua-ching. 1989. *Attune Your Body with Dao-In: Taoist Exercises for a Long and Happy Life*. Malibu, Calif.: Shrine of the Eternal Breath of Tao.

Olivelle, Patrick J. 1990. "Village vs. Wilderness: Ascetic Ideals and the Hindu World." In *Monastic Life in the Christian and Hindu Traditions,* edited by Austin B. Creel and Vasudha Narayanan, 125-60. Lewiston, NY: Edwin Mellen Press.

Robinet, Isabelle. 1984. *La révélation du Shangqing dans l'histoire du taoïsme*. 2 vols. Paris: Publications de l'Ecole Française d'Extrême-Orient.

_____. 1993. *Taoist Meditation*. Translated by Norman Girardot and Julian Pas. Albany: State University of New York Press.

Stein, Stephan. 1999. *Zwischen Heil und Heilung: Zur frühen Tradition des Yangsheng in China*. Uelzen: Medizinisch-Literarische Verlagsgesellschaft.

Strickmann, Michel. 1981. *Le taoïsme du Mao chan: chronique d'une révélation*. Paris: Collège du France, Institut des Hautes Etudes Chinoises.

Taimni, I. K. 1975. *The Science of Yoga*. Wheaton, Ill.: Theosophical Publishing House.

Wenwu 文物. 1990. "Zhangjiashan Hanjian Yinshu shiwen" 張家山漢簡引書釋文. *Wenwu* 文物 1990/10: 82-86.

Wood, Ernest. 1971. *Yoga*. Harmondsworth: Penguin.

Worthington, Vivian. 1982. *A History of Yoga*. Boston: Routlege & Kegan Paul.

Yasudian, Selvarajan, and Elizabeth Haich. 1965. *Yoga and Health*. New York: Harper & Row.

Chapter Six

Transforming Sexual Energy with

Water-and-Fire Alchemy

MICHAEL WINN

> If one abstains from intercourse,
> the spirit has no opportunity for expansiveness.
> Yin and yang are blocked and cut off from one another.
> — *Sunü jing* 素女經 [1]

Sexual love is one of the most powerful human experiences. Since ancient times, Daoists have sought to tap the power of sexuality to heal the body, to deepen love relationships, and to achieve elevated states of enlightenment. The Chinese texts on sexology are the oldest in the world, dating back about 2,300 years (Ruan 1991), and many contain question-and-answer dialogues between the Yellow Emperor and his celestial advisors or sexual consorts on how to best cultivate sexual *qi* for long life and immortality (see Cleary 1994).

The body-centered cosmology of the early sexology texts and the oral traditions of different Daoist groups have led over time to a wide spectrum of sexual practices. They include ritualized physical sexual intercourse, celibate contemplation of sexual essences copulating within the body, and conscious subtle-body love-making with a partner at a distance. Inner sexual alchemy immerses the adept in the cosmic love-making of coupled polarities in nature, such as the sun and the moon as well as planetary and starry beings (Bokenkamp 1997, 43; Wile 1992, 25; Winn 2001).

---

[1] The *Sunü jing* is the "Simple Woman's Classic," one of the key sexual manuals of ancient China. The translation follows Wile 1992, 7.

The notion that sexual energy is linked to eternal life at first glance seems counter-intuitive. The cycle of sexual birth and death defines human mortality. The idea that ephemeral sexual desires hold a hidden key to immortal life was codified by later Daoist schools of water-and-fire internal alchemy. Sexual essence or *jingqi* 精氣, is seen as the fine spiritual substance of being that can be refined into the "elixir" (*dan* 丹) of eternal life. It is the human secret to realizing the workings of the impersonal Dao, the opening and closing of its "mysterious gate."

I have personally explored these Daoist methods over the last twenty-five years as student, teacher, and experimenter, driven by an intense curiosity about the nature of sexuality, which intuitively felt central to spiritual evolution. I will share a personal Daoist sexual experience known as a "valley orgasm." But first, since the canon of Daoist sexual teachings is so huge, we need a brief overview of the basic categories of Daoist sexual practice. The first distinction is between internal and external sexual cultivation. Inner and outer alchemy practices sometimes overlap, so these are not strict divisions.

There are two kinds of external sexual cultivation (*waidan gong* 外丹 功). One branch is medical sexology which presents mostly solo cultivation methods focused on improving bodily health and relieving sexual dysfunction. They include practices using Qigong movements, self-massages, herbal prescriptions, and other medical treatments, such as massage, acupuncture, moxibustion, and the like. These medical practices generally focus on balancing the kidney and liver *qi* functions. The water phase (controlled by the kidneys) is responsible for generating sexual vitality, and the wood phase (controlled by the liver) regulates the genitals and expresses sexual *qi* (see Jarrett 1999; Dumas 1997).

The second branch of alchemy practice is the bedroom arts (*fangzhong shu* 房中術). Known popularly as dual cultivation, these "arts of the bedchamber" involve the exchange of yin and yang physical fluids and subtle essences with a sexual partner (see Wile 1992). The practices focus more on the kidney-heart relationship as the axis around which the sexual volatility of the two lovers rotates. This outer alchemical water-fire relationship needs to be understood and brought into balance before one proceeds to inner practice.

The other category of sexual practice is internal cultivation, literally "inner elixir skill" (*neidan gong* 內丹功), popularly translated as inner alchemy (see Lu 1970; Wilhelm 1962; Winn 2001). This is usually done as a meditative practice. The adept sexually couples his or her yin and yang essences internally as part of a lengthy process of defining energetic channels and opening up an inner body space or "cauldron." The adept's inner male and inner female are united within this cauldron, causing a process of spiritual rebirth. This practice is often not seen by outsiders as a sexual practice, since there is no physical sexual partner. The rarer "dual internal cultivation" practice, on the other hand, involves a pair of high-level cultivators having energetic sex (without touching) as part of their meditative practice (Liu 2001).

In the following, I will provide an overview of sexual cultivation in history and cosmology as well as the main procedures for women and men in external sexual practice for attaining immortality by copulation of water and fire.

Daoist Sexual Cultivation in History

The bedroom arts first flourished during the Han dynasty (206 B.C.E.- 220 C.E.), supported by Chinese emperors in need of skilled advisors to prevent sexual exhaustion servicing their large harem, which was their guarantee of a successor. They also sought to tap sexual love for the secret of longevity. This may account for the early Han sexology texts with conversations between female adepts and the legendary Yellow Emperor, who allegedly had 1,200 concubines.

Sex rituals also flourished during the Tang dynasty (618-907). There is some evidence that Daoist sexual practices traveled to India and stimulated the flowering of Tantric sexual practices in the sixth-seventh centuries (see Chu 1994). Internal sexual alchemy and solo meditative sexual practice achieved popularity in the Song (960-1260), while partner practice was much written about during the Ming (1368-1644) (see Liu 2001). Royal interest in sex has never flagged; when the Forbidden City was taken from the Emperor in 1911, over 1,000 sex toys were found.

In the West, Daoist sexual practices began to appear in the 1970s. They flourished as part of the sexual revolution stimulated by the psychological theories of Sigmund Freud and extended by Carl Jung, Wilhelm Reich, and Havelock Ellis. Bestselling self-improvement books—*The Joy of Sex* (Comfort 1972), *From Sex to Super Consciousness* (Rajneesh 1971), *Sexual Secrets* (Douglas and Slinger 1979), and *The Tao of Sexology* (Chang 1986)—helped fuel a new openness to sexuality that mixed Daoist and Tantric ideas, depth psychology, and the free love movement.

Western depth-psychology theory held that the sexual impulse was a fundamental shaping force of the personality. Widespread acceptance of this idea opened Westerners to the alchemical interpretation of Daoist yin-yang theory that went one step further—that sexual polarity can be transmuted into spiritual unity, that sex is the primary alchemical agent of human evolution. In his introduction to the Daoist alchemical text *Secret of the Golden Flower*, Jung tried to impose his anima-animus archetypes on yin-yang theory. He spent the last fifteen years of his life studying Western alchemy texts for their secrets. But he lacked a practical energetic methodology, beyond "talk therapy" on the couch to psychoanalyze dreams, to directly experience these subconscious male-female forces in the body and to guide them into super-conscious states (see Wilhelm 1962).

Daoist alchemical ideas attracted Jung and other Westerners because they offered practical, body-centered methods to harness the cosmic yin-yang dynamic tension underlying all male-female relations. Indian Tantra shares similar underlying principles with Daoist alchemy. But Daoist sexual practices are not as entangled with religious deities, are more practical, and offer a far more detailed subtle energetic body map. The seminal books that popularized Daoist sexology in the West were *Tao of Love and Sex* (Chang 1977) and *Taoist Secrets of Love: Cultivating Male Sexual Energy* (Winn and Chia 1984). The latter text was also translated into Chinese and has contributed to a renewed interest in Daoist sexual practices currently happening in mainland China.

Later sequels by Mantak and Maneewan Chia (1986; 1996; 2000) were reworkings of the first text, but aimed at a wider audience. These books, combined with a network of over a thousand Healing Tao teachers in thirty countries certified to teach Daoist sexual and subtle body practices, became the most visible aspect of Daoist influence in changing Western sexual paradigms. They created a major doorway for tens of thousands of Western spiritual seekers, who found themselves on a path of the previously obscure Seven Alchemy Formulas for Immortality passed on to Mantak Chia by the Daoist hermit One Cloud (Winn 2001). A more recent publication that makes Daoist sexual practice accessible to laymen was written by a couple, Mieke and Stephan Wik, telling of their experiences in distinct voices and providing easy exercises for aspiring practitioners (2005).

As practiced today, solo cultivation might begin with special breathing or Qigong practices to build up *qi* flow in the body. Stimulation arouses sexual energy, which is then circulated from either the ovaries or testicles into energy channels that flow around the body. For dual cultivation with a partner, similar procedures would be done together, with sexual massage before intercourse using special positions and coital techniques. Adepts of both solo and dual forms would likely practice Daoist meditation afterward.

Sexual Cosmology

> Dao gives birth to the One,
> One gives birth to the Two,
> Two gives birth to the Three.
> The Three give birth to the ten thousand things.
> — *Daode jing* 道德經, ch. 42 [2]

External and internal sexual alchemy, as well as solo and dual cultivation practices, all rely on the same principles of the trinity of yin-yang-*yuan*—the three stages of creation outlined in the *Daode jing*. Some Daoists only write about the two forces yin (female) and yang (male) as the most tangible aspects of nature, but Daoist alchemy presents them in a trinity including *yuan*. The cosmic yang/positive and yin/negative poles spiral and pulsate around a third pole of neutral, primordial, or original energy (*yuanqi* 元氣), which appears in the core axis of the human body as the Penetrating Vessel (*chongmai* 沖脈) that connects the top of the head to the pelvis and runs deep inside the torso. This axis cosmically extends between the formless state of pre-Heaven (*xiantian* 先天) and the physical, earthly existence of post-Heaven (*houtian* 後天). The "ten thousand things" are procreated by the copulation of Heaven and Earth, and yin-yang is their eternal multi-orgasmic movement.

Human sexual orgasm is an exquisite echo of that cosmic yin-yang pulsation. Water-and-fire alchemy is the process of interiorizing the subtle energetic love-making of the macrocosm in the microcosm of the physical body. By encouraging one's human *qi*, and especially sexual *jingqi*, to flow in rhythm and harmony with the hidden cycles

---

[2] The translation follows Ames and Hall 2003.

of nature, one's personal energy gates open to the cosmic flow of inner light and spiritual power of Dao.

The notion that yin-yang is a sexual process is widespread not only in ancient Chinese cosmological texts, but I have found it to be true in my encounters in China with modern Daoists as well. They will refer to the prime "numbers" of creation cited in chapter 42 of the *Daode jing* as commonly divided into odd or male numbers and even or female numbers that must be combined to procreate. Numbers symbolize the core yin-yang forces of nature and have a sexual polarity and a life of their own.

Mircea Eliade's *The Forge and the Crucible* (1978) offers a definitive analysis of the myths of alchemy throughout the world. He devotes an entire chapter to "The World Sexualized," showing how universally— from Africa to China—the myths of alchemical and metallurgical transmutation are a sexual process. The alchemist reaches deep into the womb of the earth to extract her precious raw gold essences, refined through a process of sexual firing and cooling.

Daoist cosmology posits the existence of a superfine formless primordial or original essence called *yuanjing* 元精. The primal yin-yang *qi*-pulsation of this essence gives birth to increasingly dense octaves of yin-yang activity, ultimately producing slowly vibrating matter on the physical plane. This continual copulation of yin-yang essence at all levels of vibration, from fast and formless to the excruciatingly slow vibration of a rock, is what gives birth to "the ten thousand things." So essentially, nature is having sex, continuously—a perpetual, nonstop orgasm. And that is why stars, planets, humans, insects, plants, and everything is bursting with this reproductive vitality.

Daoist theory details how the human process of body-creation itself is sexual. Human beings are considered a microcosm of the grand macrocosmic process of creation, so we have two levels of sexual procreation. One is external, a man and woman have sex to procreate another being, an outer child. The other is the ongoing internal process of procreating one's own body. In modern terms, it would be the eighty trillion cells in the human body dividing and birthing new cells. Basically, our normal process of existence is to internally clone ourselves.

Water-and-fire alchemy makes the energetics of that self-cloning process conscious and harnesses the internal procreative pulsation to give birth to an "inner child" that has true essence. The presence of essence is very important. It means this alchemical spiritual rebirth is not merely a passive or temporary awareness that has been birthed in meditation; it is a real, live, internally kicking baby. In Daoist oral tradition, it is described as a ball of *qi* moving around spontaneously inside the physical body, eager to grow and give birth to a new self that will eventually become a sage or immortal.

Take a moment and imagine eighty trillion cells, each one having a little mini orgasm and reproducing itself. The sound of this collective pulsating orgasmic cell activity could be described as the background hum of creation. In this case it is the hum of deep *jing* transforming itself into a tangible living body. If eighty trillion cells are sexually dividing, that is a lot of sexual activity—much richer and more potent than orgasm in the ordinary sense of the term.

Sexual Essence and Sexual Energy

The language Daoists use to talk about yin-yang orgasmic activity relies on the trinity of the Three Treasures to describe the transformations between essence (*jing* 精), subtle breath or energy (*qi* 氣), and intelligence/spirit (*shen* 神). These Three Treasures transform from one into the other, *jing* to *qi* to *shen*, and back again, *shen* to *qi* to *jing*, as one gives birth to matter and then dissolves back into spirit in each moment. Rebirthing produces a blissful state which is essentially a whole body, steady-state orgasm—powerful but unconscious in most people.

Sexual practices, from Qigong through dual cultivation to solo alchemy, are different ways to amplify and expand awareness of the flow between the two extremes of this yin-yang continuum, whole-body energetic orgasm, and physical genital orgasm. They are two ways of looking at the same process, but happening at different vibrational speeds. Simply becoming aware that the body is having internal sex on a cellular level can relieve feelings of sexual frustration or energize someone who is sick and depleted.

In Chinese medicine, the term "kidneys" indicates a broad energetic sphere that includes the sexual organs, kidneys, urinary bladder, and their various meridians. In men, this includes the penis, testicles, and prostate gland; in women, the ovaries, vagina, uterus, and breasts. The kidneys' inherent intelligence regulates the endocrine glands, brain, blood, bone marrow, and sexual essence, all fundamental to long life. But we need to be clear: "Kidneys" in Chinese medicine is not the same as the physical kidneys of Western medicine. It does not mean just the two bean-shaped organs which are quite tiny, smaller than a fist, even though they have a big job to do. In classical Chinese medicine, "kidneys" designates a sphere of influence that penetrates and regulates the biological, psychological, and spiritual functions of the water phase. Kidney-water is the most latent and foundational among the five phases, associated with winter, darkness, and the north. It is responsible for birthing everything.

Jing, the subtle essence governed by the kidneys holds the shape patterns of the body. *Jing* is the key ingredient to apprehending the function of sexuality. *Jing* is perhaps best understood in Western terms as prime energy, the raw fuel that drives the pulsating rhythm of the body's moment-to-moment cellular division and reproduction of itself. In modern terms, *jing* generates stem cells, genes, and the sexual hormonal energy of the glands, but is not sexual energy itself.

Jing in humans is governed by a psycho-biological aspect of kidney water called *zhi* 志, literally the "will." *Zhi* is the instinctual will to be embodied, to survive, to seek pleasure, and to fulfill a specific destiny while in a body. It controls the *jing* that in the human animal is radi-

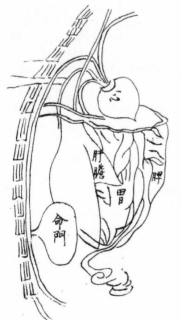

ating polarized waves of male or female sexed energy which we may label charisma or magnetic power. In short, *jing* is the raw source of sexual desire and the feeling essence of earthiness, while *zhi* is the instinctive intelligence that governs the unfolding of *jing*.

Without *jing,* the heart and its psycho-biological aspect, spirit (*shen* 神), would not be able to embody its virtues or have direct sensory experience of physicality (see Fig. 1). If one is feeling "spiritual bliss," the bliss part is the feeling of smoothly vibrating *jing,* perceived with the lens of the heart and the other vital organs. This *jing-shen* relationship between the kidneys and the heart can be volatile, *jing* often being the main source of vexation for spiritual seekers who ignore it or run from their sexual impulses in order to chase after

Fig. 1. The energetic connections between the heart and kidneys.

the other end of the spectrum of consciousness, the heart-spirit. Combining kidneys and heart is the local portal of self-awareness which integrates with the other body spirits to become the "great spirit," an infinite sea of pure awareness. To achieve the state of great spirit, the seeker must ground his or her heart-spirit in the essence of kidney-*jing*.

What, then, is the difference between *jing* as essence and *jingqi* as sexual energy? *Jing* holds the infrastructure of the bodily form together and is stored in the bone marrow, where blood and hormonal precursors are manufactured before moving into the endocrine glands and blood vessels. In Chinese medicine, *jing* has a function similar to what Western medicine calls the stem cells. It represents a primal force that differentiates into many functions. A stem cell, like *jing,* can become a heart cell or a kidney cell, a skin cell or a brain cell, or whatever it needs to become. According to Chinese medical theory, we basically manufacture ourselves in the bones and the brain marrow, which is also known as the Ocean of Essence (*jinghai* 精海).

This deep sea of *jing* in the brain, bones, and the Penetrating Vessel emanates the *jingqi* of sexual practice that then flows in all the meridians. This relation does not exist for Western sexologists who define sexual energy purely in terms of physiological response. They know that when someone gets sexually excited there is more blood flow, the heart is beating a little faster, there may be increased hormonal activity. Testosterone or estrogen levels change. There are tumescence, genital swelling, an erection, or vaginal swelling to increase friction, and also a swelling against certain nerves. That is as much as Western sexologists recognize. They do not see an energetic network or the connection of sexual energy to marrow.

In contrast, the Chinese distinguish at least thirty-three types of *qi* in the major meridians, not to mention hundreds of divergent and sinew meridians. Sexual or *jingqi* is one of them, yet it is also very different from them. Unlike them, it has a sticky quality that allows it to act as the stabilizing or bonding energy between opposing female-male or yin-yang forces. This stickiness is the reason why it is so difficult to separate from a sexual partner and why divorce is frequently such a struggle. Sexual energy not only creates attachment to other bodies, but glues itself to emotions, thoughts, perceptions of identity, and the like. Thus, to maintain an energetic equilibrium it is essential that the mind remains calm and unattached during sexual practice. As the medical classic *Huangdi neijing suwen* 黃帝內經素問 (The Yellow Emperor's Inner Classic, Simple Questions) says:

As for the way to engage in sexual intercourse, calmness
makes for strength. Make the mind as calm as water, con-
serve the spiritual dew within. Knock at the jade gate with
the jade stalk, the mind neither too tense nor too loose. You
can tell what is best by how the woman sighs in response.
Collect the spiritual mist, drink the celestial broth, sending
them to the internal organs in order to store them deeply.
(Cleary 1994, 20)

Five Organ Forces Nourished by Sex

Jingqi has the power to amplify or multiply whatever it bonds to. It
intensifies emotions, thoughts, and sensations; it multiplies cell and
glandular reproduction rates, either within the body or by giving
birth to children. It can also be directed to amplify creative energy in
the world of play or career so that, wherever people focus our sexual
energy, it multiplies into abundance. Sexual energy thus acts as a
bonding agent between the different layers of the energy body on the
continuum between *jing*, *qi*, and *shen*. It cycles through the body's
five phases as they move along the productive cycle.

While the five major organs with their inherent bio-psychological
forces function separately, at a deep level they remain one, and thus
can function simultaneously in harmony with each other. The productive cycle of the five phases flows from water to wood to fire to earth
to metal. In the body this translates into a cycle flowing from kidneys
to liver to heart to spleen to lungs. If *qi*-flow is healthy, each organ
will add to the vitality of the next organ in the cycle. As the *Yufang
bijue* 玉房秘訣 (Secrets of the Jade Chamber) says:

To improve the functioning of the five organs, facilitate digestion, and cure the hundred ills, wait for the approach of
ejaculation, then expand your belly and mentally move the
qi around the body. Next, contract your belly again so that
the *jing* disperses and reverts to the hundred vessels. Then
penetrate your partner nine times shallow and once deeply
between her zither strings and grain ears. Good *qi* will return, ill *qi* will depart. (Wile 1992, 104)

The exercise activates the sexual energy in the cycle of the five
phases, beginning with the kidneys and their *jingqi*. If sexual energy
is strong here, the next phase, represented by the liver and its force,
the celestial soul (*hun* 魂), are nourished and start to expand the *jing*
to the rest of the body. Blood flow begins to quicken and excitement

arises. The liver stores blood and uses it to regulate the arousal of the genitals, controlling the blood flow needed for an erection. It activates the tendons and sends blood to the muscles, which translates into the passionate movement of grasping one's lover during intercourse.

Third in the cycle is the heart with its force of the spirit. Its feeling of love and joy may amplify the sexual energy and project it out romantically to another person—or alternatively to the whole cosmos as divine love. The heart-fire warms the *jingqi* further and raises its vibration into a feeling of whole-body radiance.

Following this, the earth phase, manifest in the spleen and the intention (*yi* 意), stabilizes and grounds the love-making process. That is to say, sexual love opens up one's inner space or "inner earth" to trusting one's lover. The private inner space of each person becomes a shared collective inner space. Practitioners share the inner "earth" of their being with their lover because the intention that governs our sense of trust and intimacy is strengthened by love-making. It controls our sense of boundary, and sexuality is about exploring and dissolving physical boundaries. Physically, the *jingqi* at this stage infuses the flesh to become especially sensitive. The mouth and lips, the body opening of the spleen and stomach, will begin to kiss more deeply and perhaps fiercely.

Lastly, the metal phase is linked to the lungs and the corporeal soul (*po* 魄). It regulates *jingqi* through the breath and controls the amount of *qi* that breath brings into the love-making. An orgasm in the lungs during love-making might take the form of temporarily stopping the breath. This means the lung-*po* is ecstatic and breathes only internal *qi*. It also brings in a sense of the personal, expressed commonly in the question: "How does this sexual relation strengthen my identity?" The metal aspect of the lungs is the most evolutionary of the five phases as it can melt into liquid, take any form, and hold individual shape for as long as necessary. It is also a metaphor for the alchemical journey of the personal self and the need to refine our inner *qi* into spiritual gold, i.e. into an incorruptible and immortal state.

Thus we can see how sexual energy can be circulated in the postnatal creation cycle to strengthen both our biological and psychological selves. The vital organs with their various forces control energy flow in the meridians, and feel refreshed and recharged by the vibrant yin-yang pulsation of sexual energy. The fire of the heart and the water of the kidneys are the most volatile, and thus are given the most importance in sexual alchemy. Water and fire stimulate each other and keep the other in check. By maintaining a proper exchange between them, one enters a steady state that gradually opens the door to more refined love-making. Simply keeping an open heart, one protects against blind lust, which ultimately injures the kidneys because it can never be satisfied by physical sex alone. All aloneness at its core, the heart-spirit seeks the love, sensual touch, and sexual stimulation of the kidneys. The mirror of this loneliness is the embodied kidney-will seeking the heart's spiritual virtue of unconditional acceptance and love.

Women's Practice

> You should know that the desire of women is stronger than that of men. Once the monthly flow stops, her heart is like a blossoming lotus bud. It benefits from rain and dew and begins to grow its fruit.
>
> A woman without a man is yin in isolation– she cannot bring forth a lotus blossom. Unless she receives the benefit of rain and dew, she is like a field without manure: useless.
> – *Nüdan yaoyan* 女丹要言[3]

Women face two main challenges when cultivating sexual energy. One is the physical depletion of *jing* that occurs naturally due to their monthly cycle. The cure for this is found in practices that lighten or eliminate the loss of blood during menstruation through dietary adjustments, meditations, and self massages. The other challenge is the natural tendency of the uterus to contract. Under emotional stress, this may lead to an excessive or chronic contraction and thus cause *qi* stagnation in the sexual organs.

A women's ovaries store tremendous creative power, potentially available for bearing children but also ready to enhance internal biological health. Daoist alchemical practice taps this female *jing* for spiritual rebirth. However, any suppressed emotional and sexual energy in the uterus can block the natural pathways of revitalizing the energy flow and may cause psychic exhaustion. It may result in pre-menstrual syndrome, ovarian or uterine cysts, and eventually cause some form of chronic illness.

---

[3] A text on women's practice from the eighteenth century, this title translates "Key Words on Women's Alchemy." The translation follows Despeux and Kohn 2003, 212.

Women have some natural advantages over men in overcoming the challenge of harmonizing their sexual energy. Their breasts function as an extra motor in the body, like an extra set of "upper kidneys" that provide more kidney power. This is needed for bearing children and breast-feeding—the latter being energetically more exhausting then pregnancy because mother's milk is blood converted into milk. The breast-feeding mother must constantly replace her blood, which taxes her kidneys and thus her *jing*. To do so, she is equipped with a second pair of essence-producing organs.

A second factor giving superior sexual strength to a woman is that the biological location of her sexual organs is more internal. This causes sexual energy to be spontaneously circulated in the meridians, stored in the vital organs, and expressed through the personality. It may also explain why many women seem to have a stronger—and more volatile—emotional life than men. This is the yang or fiery power hidden within their yin or watery nature, a fundamental concept of Daoist alchemy. If the volatile water and fire mixture underlying a woman's emotional and sexual life are not harmonized, the result will be expressed through swings in biological and emotional processes.

A third factor contributing to the superior sexual strength of women is their abundant supply of pre-natal *jing* in the unfertilized eggs in the ovaries. Of course the ancients had no way to count these eggs, which modern science has revealed to number in the hundreds of thousands, far more than needed for childbirth. But Daoists have traditionally held that women have a nearly infinite supply of yin-energy due to their strong sexual potential, and this yin-potential can be converted into manifesting yang for spiritual growth.

However, in many cases the yin-potential is locked up because the uterus is packed with trapped emotional and sexual *qi*. This blockage is a kind of excessive earth-centered gravity in women. It is a yin virtue in that it leads them to develop strong nurturing and cooperative qualities. Daoist wisdom holds that even though women have a natural sexual-spiritual advantage, their deep and often excessive uterine-earth contraction makes it far more difficult for women to open the core channel of the Penetrating Vessel. They find it hard to spiritually ascend their essence to rebirth their spirit in the upper elixir field in the head, the spiritual gateway to Heaven.

The combination of ovary power and a dual set of kidneys gives women an inherently stronger sexual nature than men. This is why many male sexual practices are designed in part to balance out that inequality. Men have the compensation of a simpler energetic system and an easier time of opening the core channel, as they have no uterus in which to contract their *qi*. In men, the *jingqi* follows a different pathway, and is more likely to get stuck in the head.

It must also be kept in mind that women are constantly resonating with a completely different natural cycle than men. Women's blood is governed by a deep earth cycle, reflected in the lunar cycle of their menses. Resonance with the moon and its pull on blood and sexual energy further nourishes female kidney strength. The moon functions like a giant kidney in its regulation of the water phase on earth. The lunar and earth influence implies a slower watery female cycle, rather than the fiery, hot daily solar male cycle. This naturally creates a lot of potential complications in communications and relationships between men and women.

Women lose *jing* through excessive bleeding during the releasing half of the menstrual cycle. By energetically detoxifying the body with sexual Qigong during the building half of the cycle, the need for bleeding as a means of detoxifying is vastly reduced. Circular breast massage, Ovarian Breathing, and Slaying the Red Dragon are the primary methods for regulating cyclical hormonal fluctuations, made more powerful by inner alchemy meditation.

An example of such an alchemical meditation is the internal circulation of female *jingqi* in the microcosmic orbit, which in most texts—written by male adepts—flows along the fire path, moving from the perineum up the spine, over the crown of the head, and down the water path, i.e., from the lower lip through the center of the chest to the navel. It regulates yin-yang balance in all meridians and opens energetic communication between the endocrine glands situated along the orbit: the reproductive gonads, adrenal, pituitary, pineal, thyroid, para-thyroid, and pancreas glands, plus the spleen and heart, organs that often behave like glands.

More appropriately, the orbit for women may flow more easily in the reverse direction, moving up the water path along the Conception Vessel from the perineum through the chest to the mouth and, after moving across the head, descending along the fire path of the Governing Vessel along the spine back to the perineum. This is known as "water leading fire." Which direction of flow is chosen is best determined by body type and spontaneous openness to inner communication. However, women during and after menopause are cautioned to lead with the water path, and it may help to moderate hot flashes.

After conservation of blood is achieved, women progress to the cultivation of ovarian essence. For women practicing dual cultivation, this includes absorbing male sexual essence and redirection of the genital orgasm to the spine, chest, heart, and into the vital organs until full body orgasm is achieved. Because the female breast/water-heart/fire relationship stabilizes the *jing* in the middle elixir field and because of the more internal location of the vagina, ovaries, and uterus, internal recirculation of sexual energy is somewhat easier for women than for men. This may account for women finding it easier to achieve multi-orgasmic sexual experiences.

Further distinction for external sexual alchemy cultivators can be made between clitoral and vaginal orgasm. Clitoral orgasm is more fiery as it is linked to the liver complex that controls the nervous system and feeds the heart fire. Vaginal orgasm is considered to be more whole body, due to the zones of reflexology within the vagina that reflect the stimulation of the entire five phase cycle that cause the *jingqi* to "enter the hundred vessels" and thus heal all illness.

In ancient times the heart was considered the natural center for women; it expressed the center of gravity of their heart fire, balanced between two watery breasts. Modern women have become more similar to men, being much more active in the outer world and thus more yang. In the Chinese Qigong community, the modern trend toward equal functions for men and women has been noted and held responsible for modern women's center of gravity shifting down to the navel center from the heart center. A sample view of this shift was found among four female adepts in China I have spoken with in recent years. A Daoist nun on Mount Hua summarized the view I heard elsewhere: "I begin cultivating in the lower elixir field. After that is open, I shift up to my heart center and practice from there. I invite the spirit of the Queen Mother of the West to enter my heart and guide me."

A more physical sexual cultivation technique for women is to exercise their vaginal muscles by inserting a jade egg into their vagina and move it about as an internal exercise. This method was introduced to Mantak Chia as part of the oral tradition he received. The physical exercise aids women in restoring sexual function and tightening stretched vaginal tissue after childbirth. It also seals the Meeting of Yin (Huiyin 會陰, CV-1) point at the perineum against leakage of *qi* caused by excess sitting. The movement of the jade egg is a solo practice for stimulating the internal sexual reflexology points that activate the flow of *qi* to the five vital organs. Quiet sitting with the egg in state of deep stillness allows the egg to be used as a medium for absorbing psychic toxins trapped in the uterus (Piontek 2001). This practice has become popular among Western female sexual energy cultivators. Because most of the ancient sexology practices have gone underground in communist China, it is difficult to know if this practice continues there today.

The medical applications of female sexual practice include relief of pre-menstrual syndrome and menopausal hot flashes, healing of infertility ("cold womb syndrome") and a variety of glandular and sexual dysfunctions, including frigidity. Some Western women have completely stopped their menstrual cycle through voluntary internal practice. Most use it to simply lighten the amount and color of blood flow as they learn how to detoxify their blood. An important aspect of Daoist sexual practices for Western women is the sense of empowerment it offers. It is part of the larger paradigm shift of women gaining greater control over their inner sexual forces and seemingly immutable cycles of menstruation (see Chia and Chia 1986).

Male Attainment

> The way to extend life involves watching over the closing off of the flow of semen. When the semen is locked up and stored in a timely manner, then spiritual clarity comes and builds up.
>
> When it builds up, it inevitably becomes evident. Locking up the semen to stabilize vitality (*jing*) ensures that the supply of sexual fluid is never exhausted. Then diseases do not affect you . . . and you can live to be one hundred years old.
> — *Sunü jing*

Men are on a much shorter cycle than women: the reproduction of sperm only takes twenty-four hours. Once a man has ejaculated, on this short cycle he may want to release it again the next day. Sperm is the male storehouse of *jingqi*—lost through excessive sex and ejaculation. Modern science offers some confirming evidence—a single ejaculation may cost a male between 300 to 500 million spermatozoa, which could be used for rejuvenation through Daoist methods. A scientific study showed that male nematode worms lived twice as long when they were altered to prevent sperm loss. The conclusion: constant production of sperm taxes the male biologically (Angier 1992).

The Daoist definition of "excessive" ejaculation varies according to body type, age, and climate. Ejaculation has less immediate impact on a healthy young male because of his abundance of *jing*. But all men must be especially careful during the winter, when kidney-*qi* moves inward rather than out. In spring, it is healthy to ejaculate more since the liver-*qi* is trying to expand outwards. There are methods of slowing down ejaculation during sex, so that men can draw out the essence from their sperm and recycle it around the body to nourish other energy centers. These practices include Testicle Breathing and Drawing Up the Golden Nectar, a method of internally sucking sexual *jingqi* up the spine as if it were liquid in a straw.

This technique, also called "reverting sexual energy to nourish the brain" (*huanjing bunao* 還精補腦), has been known in Daoist literature for the past two thousand years (Skar and Pregadio 2000, 467; Wile 1992). It may well have begun as a sexual practice to rejuvenate the brain and evolved to become a spiritual practice as the *qi* was observed to spiral up the spine and down the chest, blending the fire and water *qi* of the body and eventually causing the spirit to crystallize in the lower elixir field. Today the practice of circulating *qi* around the body is a famous meditation known as the microcosmic orbit. It creates a transitional pathway for *qi*-flow between external and internal sexual alchemy, between cultivating post-natal and pre-natal *qi* (see Chia 1983).

It is not necessary to become celibate to gain the benefits of recycling sexual energy for purposes besides reproduction. Celibacy is often the intent to sublimate sexual desire into a religious goal (see Eskildsen 1998). Daoist sexual energy cultivation with a partner (or solo, through masturbation) allows one to satisfy the need for sexual pleasure without sacrificing male life energy to the demands of constant sperm production. The Daoist methods of conserving seed essences simultaneously transmute that essence into internal spiritual processes.

The goal of external sexual alchemy accordingly is to shift from a limited genital orgasm to a whole-body orgasm. Slowing or stopping ejaculation does not prevent a man from having orgasm or being multi-orgasmic. Ejaculation is the physical release of sexual fluid caused by a mini-orgasm in the prostate gland, which pumps the semen so it has enough momentum to enter deep into the female uterus. It also adds a clear fluid that supplies nutrition to the sperm for their journey to the egg that it hopes has ripened and is waiting on the wall of the uterus.

From the viewpoint of Daoist sexology, orgasm is defined by the pulsation of sexual energy and is not to be confused with ejaculation, which releases seed essence out the "ancestral muscle" or "jade stalk." Intensification and circulation of sexual *qi* can cause the rest of the meridians and organs to pulsate in unison. But men must stay relaxed, and not get obsessed with stopping ejaculation. The danger for beginners holding their seed is that they may also stop the *qi* pulsation at the root of orgasm. What works best is to focus on opening up the *qi*-channels and redirecting and recycling sexual *qi* before, during, and after orgasm.

In this way, ejaculation is delayed while other energy centers, vital organs, and meridians are absorbing the circulating sexual energy. Then, as the *qi* has already largely been extracted from the semen, physical ejaculation does not cause major loss of *qi*. Delaying ejaculation also allows the man to slow down his fire to stay in closer harmony with the woman's slower water cycle of arousal. This is known as "pairing the fire to match the water." It is a practical way for men to solve the common problem of premature ejaculation. A combination of continuous Testicle Breathing and sexual foreplay to "warm the woman's stove" allow the male to match the longer female lovemaking cycle. With practice a gradual shift is made from external to internal alchemy. The short-lived genital orgasm transitions into a blissful, steady whole-body orgasm that pulses all organs and meridians. When this faster vibrating pulsation becomes conscious in the deeper Eight Extraordinary Vessels and the three elixir fields, the practitioner experiences what can be described as a spiritual orgasm.

Innumerable other external methods support the sexual cultivation process. One is Tongue Gongfu for strengthening that versatile sexual muscle; another is a method for absorbing *qi* directly into the genitals from the sun. Ancient texts mention that hiding of the sexual organs under clothing leads to their disuse, which may cause early death. Men can balance their excess yang-*qi* by mixing it with yin-*qi* drawn up from the earth. This cools and grounds the hot male sexual fire and supports the body's absorption of sexual *qi* for the purpose of self-healing.

For both sexes, Daoist medical sexology posits that poor diet, shallow breathing, negative emotions and bad mental attitudes exhaust sexual vitality as quickly as semen or blood loss. Improving these with a regular meditation and Qigong practice for least twenty minutes a day is key to preventing low sexual energy and many associated dysfunctions.

The Yin-Yang of Sexual Relationships

Between the two basic Daoist approaches to achieving sexual equilibrium, the external or dual cultivation requires finding a sexual partner and forming a deep dyadic relationship (see Fig. 2). It may appear that this exchange involves only the two poles of yin-yang, between one woman and one man. However, the Daoist cultivator quickly finds out that sex involves not just two polarities, but rather four. Regardless of one's sexual preference, each person has an inner male or an inner female. One half identifies with the physical body and creates sexual identity as outer male or female; the other half is hidden in the shadow of the psyche but may dominate sexual preferences. Since both partners have an inner male or inner female, that doubles the energetic complexity. There are now four sexual identities influencing the relationship, with the possibility of four different sexual agendas.

Most men and women play out these polar roles and exchange sexual energy in a way that hopefully creates equilibrium. This is where cultivating inner stillness, the hallmark of the third pole of original *qi* in addition to yin and yang, becomes essential to holding one's center of a relationship in the midst of complexity. If the relationship becomes stable and love is present, the couple may spontaneously build up *qi*, expressed as a common shared center of stillness.

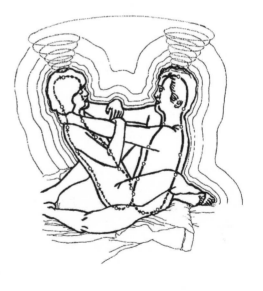

Fig. 2: Yin-yang sexual energy exchange

This is most often seen in long-term couples who are content to merely sit in the presence of each other with no need to stimulate or complete the other in any particular way. Their relationship has become a container for the neutral force at the core of their yin-yang dynamic. In religious language, sharing of this original *qi* could be called divine love, as it is grounded in a field that goes beyond sex and emotion.

Spiritual bonding is what ultimately holds human love together; it makes sexual love into a sacred art. The ability to go beyond polarity into the non-dual state of inner stillness shared with another makes sex feel sacrosanct. Relations in the beginning may only be held together by emotions, words, demonstrations of affection, and yin-yang attraction on the sexual level. But ultimately there has to be some deeper internal energetic glue, as the initial yin-yang attraction at the *jing*-level is satisfied and begins to fade. Then the attraction is sustained by refining the yin-yang polarities at deeper levels of energy, spirit, and the supreme mystery of Dao. In Western terms, this refinement process progresses from body through personality to a core sense of authentic being and cosmic consciousness.

From the Daoist view of dual cultivation, the hidden purpose of any long-term commitment is to help each other grow in original nature— ultimately a spiritual purpose. People ostensibly stay together for all kinds of reasons, including economics, social pressure, fear of change, obligation to children, or mere habit. However, underneath all these there may well be a deeper reason, which according to Daoism is that we can continue to create something together through the interaction of yin and yang energies and can reach an equilibrium in which original *qi* can manifest itself.

Inner Sexual Alchemy of Water and Fire

> The life-force of the valley never dies —
> This is called the dark female.
> The gateway of the dark female —
> This is called the root of the world.
> Wispy and delicate, it only seems to be there,
> Yet its productivity is bottomless.
> —*Daode jing*, ch. 6

The sexual fertility expressed in this image of a cosmic female vagina highlights the connection between cosmology and sexuality found in the ancient Daoist classic. Nature is experienced by the sage who is in touch with Dao as a continuous cosmic orgasm. Dao sexually births physical creation through the pulsating yin-yang process arising from primordial *qi*. The sexual nature of the original state of chaos-unity (*hundun* 混沌)— from which the ten thousand things arise and to which they eventually return—was the basis for Daoist cultivation of human sexual energy in order to return to the origin (see Tortchinov 1997).

The outer sexual methods strengthen the body and balance the mind, but here fire and water rarely come to full completion. Outer male fire and outer female water temporarily satisfy each other through sexual intercourse. But this is illusory, the postnatal fire-and-water *qi* build up their sexual charge again, seeking for another experience. *Qi* from a genital orgasm will disperse. This pattern will continue until the sexual seeker is finally fatigued by the chase, or sexual energy is effectively spent and no longer drives the individual.

In this context, people naturally ask: why is there such friction between men and women? Why is not life a joyful dance of playful opposites that accumulates more energy? In Daoist view, why does false or excess yin-yang usurp a true yin-yang dynamic? Why does it turn possessive, angry, violent, and soul-shattering at times? Partly it results from the frustration of chasing after post-natal *qi*—sexual and otherwise—that does not last. But there is a deeper reason.

The outer sexual tension between men and women is also a reflection of tension between the inner masculine and inner feminine aspects hidden within most people. The same dynamic tension that exists between our becoming—our sexualized body essence—and our formless being also flows into our relationships. The horizontal social-sexual tension is a reflection of the vertical Heaven-Earth tension. It is ultimately the tension between our outer and inner selves, our mortal and immortal ways of being.

Sexual inner alchemy is a method for peeling off the layers of yin-yang imbalance protecting us from experiencing our original innate self beyond this dynamic. What is the likely cosmic cause of this false yin-yang tension? Daoist texts allude to a "golden age" that preceded our physical existence. Study of the alchemical process, whose primary goal is to cultivate primordial *qi* in the physical body, allows an educated speculation. Many layers of psychic stress may have resulted from the tear in the fabric of the life force when the androgynous prenatal self was polarized into physical male and female bodies in postnatal existence. The androgynous self had both male-female poles within its body and was self-regenerating, or immortal. Its yin-yang cycle of life and death was renewed at will by drawing on the third force, the primordial *qi* (see Girardot 1983).

The fall into physically sexed bodies was a fall into mortality. The original qi of harmonized yin and yang was scattered by the splitting of the sexes. So when we alchemically work on resolving the yin-yang sexual tension within ourselves, and gathering the stillness of the primordial within, we are by resonance also working on the sexual wound that exists within the collective psyche of humanity from this male-female split.

Understanding of this inner yin-yang dynamic highlights the fundamental difference between external sexual alchemy and inner sexual alchemy. Outer methods involve skillful management of sexual fluids and energy to improve physical health and to harmonize a sexual relationship with a partner or with one's own sexed body. The inner sexual methods focus on using sexual polarity to accelerate the unfolding of the human spirit. Completing one's sexual identity at the deepest level fulfills both our worldly destiny (ming 命) and our spiritual inner nature (xing 性). The first stage is to awaken and rebirth our sexed body into a pure androgynous (bi-sexed or yin-yang balanced) energy body of golden light. This light or energy body is essential to consciously integrating our sexual essence with our pre-sexual self.

What makes human life so sexually confusing is that we have present at each moment three different sexual impulses influencing our consciousness: a male or female physical self, a male-female subtle energetic self, and an asexual primal spiritual self. Merging with Dao ultimately requires the integration of these three seemingly separate identities. Their interaction in the body mirrors the flow of qi in Daoist cosmogony: human qi evolves through primordial, prenatal, and postnatal stages. From the last, from Earth, we must cultivate our sexually polarized yin and yang qi to return back to the origin.

How is this practically accomplished? Inner alchemy captures the subtle polarized forces of the cosmos and internalizes them within the energy body of the adept. An inner alchemy adept becomes spiritually pregnant, conceives an immortal embryo, gives birth to an inner immortal child who, with spiritual nurturing, matures into a sage or celestial immortal—hopefully within one lifetime (see Fig. 3). All this happens while still in a physically sexed body. The function of this inner sage is to harmonize the creation of body and personality and to orchestrate fulfillment of the ultimate mission. The sage is the cosmic pattern embodied and empowered with an inner will independent of the outer world. He has a life beyond physical death, and thus he is immortal; he lives in multiple dimensions, whereas before there is a human "monkey mind": an un-integrated sea of outer wills floating about, grasping after physical straws.

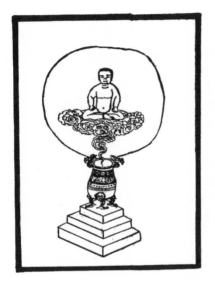

Alchemy uses simple sexual metaphors to describe progressive states of enlightenment and spiritual immortality. Every stage of alchemy refines our sexual essence and marries it to a higher level of spirit. This inner pairing of water and fire cultivates the continuation of individuated consciousness after death—but attempts to fully penetrate that mystery while the adept is still alive.

Fig. 3: The immortal embryo emerges from the alchemical cauldron.

Valley Orgasm

How, then, does inner water-and-fire alchemy impact on the sexual experience of the practitioner? The short answer is that it creates orgasmic waves of increasingly powerful subtle body pulsations through the blissful coupling of one's sexual kidney essence and one's heart spirit (see Wik and Wik 2005). Body as water and heart as fire are in an ongoing, sexually polarized primal relationship. Their coupling manifests in a more tangible, subtle energy body which mediates between the physical body and the heart's field of spiritual awareness. Sexual essence is what allows us to give substance and tangible experience to our inner being.

All this may seem impossibly abstract from the ordinary perspective of a male or female ego-sexed mind. So I offer a description of a Daoist "valley orgasm," experienced in 1984 by myself and my partner who is now my wife (see Winn and Chia 1984). The most interesting point of this and numerous other experiences of subtle-body and at-a-distance spirit sex is that they usually *precede* the act of physical love-making, i.e. they are not caused by physical intercourse. Rather the physical intercourse which may or may not follow is mostly a way to ground and digest the cosmic forces experienced:

> Joyce and I removed our clothes. We sat cross-legged on the bed facing each other, naked. It was our intent to meditate before making love. We both did testicle or ovarian breathing and circulated the sexual energy in the orbit to harmonize our sexual feelings in our three elixir fields. We each smiled to our inner heart, deep in the body's core. There was no visualization or attempt to create any experience—we were simply in a state of naked surrender to each other. In deep silence, we noticed that a new and unusual pulsation began to envelop us.
>
> It felt to me like a simultaneous yin and yang orgasm. The yang orgasm was my energy body pulsing with Joyce's, expanding out in waves, that became inconceivably vast. We zoomed faster than the speed of light past planets and galaxies and then ecstatically merged into formless swirls of light and sound. The yang orgasm kept exploding out beyond our bodies.
>
> The yin orgasm was an equal and opposite implosion deep within our bodies. Some powerful gravitational vortex kept sucking us into a tiny point that was incredibly heavy. I could feel that Joyce was inside that point as well. I felt deeply embodied and centered within my personal self.
>
> The yin and yang orgasm was a marriage of sexual counterforces. They held the space for a neutral observer in us to perfectly experience both orgasmic feelings at once. We sat in this state for half an hour, amazed and dumbfounded. It finally subsided. We fell into each others arms, knowing that a great and sacred mystery had been revealed to us. Our love-making was lovely and tender, but somehow anticlimatic. The shared yin-yang orgasm is what we remember, it is forever seared into our souls, and impelled us to marry.
>
> This valley orgasm permanently shifted the nature of our sexual relationship. Our subtle bodies would quickly attune and later we found we could exchange deep sexual energy for hours, lying beside each other, naked or clothed, without any physical stimulation or intercourse. It was a direct exchange of our sexed subtle bodies. As our energy bodies mingled and coupled, we were infused with loving spiritual qualities. This led to long periods of spontaneous abstention from physical intercourse that could last for many months,

but with exquisitely sublime daily subtle body coitus. As our subtle bodies crystallized and became more "real," we eventually graduated to astral sex—the ability to intentionally exchange orgasmic subtle energy at great distances.

Daoist cultivators often experience profound shifts in their sexual identity when they first move from external to internal alchemy. Their primal fire-and-water *qi* is focused in a very deep inner space within the body. This inner copulation can temporarily cause a loss of outer sexual desire. Eventually, the energy body re-organizes itself and begins to operate from this new inner space, which produces true or authentic yin or yang sexual energy. This changes the biological, psychological, and spiritual levels of one's sexual identity. Sexual drive returns after some months, but with a major difference: sex is no longer a compulsory-habitual sex drive.

Sexual attraction becomes a choice, a deeply centered response to someone, but is no longer an unconscious biological instinct coming from his or her genitals. Adepts have shifted deeper inside the body and merged their spirit and essence; thus their inner male and female dynamic becomes conscious. The birth of a new androgynous "spiritual embryo" means they have opened a third and more neutral perspective on sexual polarity, rather than endless unconscious struggles for power between their male and female aspects that is acted out or projected onto other people.

Conclusion

The tension between resting in pure being and becoming a sexual body is so powerful that most enlightenment states rarely resolve this duality. Proof is seen in the uncontrolled sexual behavior of numerous self-described "enlightened" teachers from many different meditation traditions (Winn 2002a). Daoist sexual alchemy attempts to go beyond meditative quieting of the postnatal mind and breath by coupling and internalizing within the body the many subtle levels of yin-yang sexual tension that exist in the cosmos. It offers a practical body-centered process that step by step builds a harmonic bridge between the tiny, slow vibration of our individual human heartbeat and sexual essence and the cosmic inner heart in whirling galaxies, black holes, and vast formless dimensions.

Sex drive, essential to the survival of any species, is also the driving force in humanity's spiritual evolution. Resolving sexual tension is the unconscious impetus behind religious seeking to return to an asexual, formless divine state with unconditioned spiritual qualities. Daoist sexual alchemy is thus a progressive pairing of water and fire at the physical and spirit levels of our sexual identity. Its premise is that the universe is sexed, and we need to understand male-female sexuality in relation to subtle sexual forces hidden within nature.

Humanity's central spiritual task is to resolve its mortal sexual tension, which creates the fear of death at the root of most sickness and social ills. Sexual alchemy speeds human awareness of the relation between all yin-yang polarities to immortal cosmic *qi*. Healing humanity's deep and divisive sexual wound is synonymous with repairing a deep tear in the yin-yang fabric of the life force.

The ultimate goal of Daoist sexual alchemy is to restore communication with our immortal, nondual, pre-sexual being. But it is not practical to go directly from living in a sexed body to being a no-sexed entity without repressing the sexual drive. A way must be found for them to co-exist. In reality even an enlightened human being remains physically sexed. The alchemical solution is to grow an energy body with both poles, male and female, in deep functional harmony.

This bi-sexed androgynous energy body acts as a go-between of our physical body and core spiritual self. The energy body gradually becomes the central identity. Alchemical formulas help us to absorb within the physical body the macrocosmic yin-yang of sun, moon, planets, and stars needed to make a vibrational shift into universal consciousness. Once the energy body becomes stable, i.e., a true body and not merely a mental or astral projection, our pre-sexual spiritual self can consciously function within the sexed physical plane. This constitutes a complete journey from creation back to origin. This is not a regression into a primal or primitive state; the second half of that journey from primordiality back into creation requires the integration of our primal self with our sexual and socialized self.

Following Dao is ultimately about diving into the state before creation, the supreme mystery of life, and emerging fresh, reborn. Daoists seek a conscious relationship with the life force and the source from which it arises. We mostly act out our desire for this ultimate mystery of the unified state before creation with the more manageable, small sexual mystery of loving another person. By opening our hearts and entering the dark sexual mystery hidden inside own body, we are also able to directly merge with Dao.

Bibliography

Ames, Roger, and Hall, David. 2003. *Dao De Jing: A Philosophical Translation*. New York: Ballantine.

Angier, Natalie. 1992. "In Worm, Making Sperm is Found to Shorten a Male's Life." *New York Times* 12-3, 1992.

Bokenkamp, Stephen. 1997. *Early Daoist Scriptures*. Berkeley: University of California Press.

Chang, Jolan. 1977. *Tao of Love and Sex*. New York: Dutton.

Chang, Stephen. 1986. *The Tao of Sexology: The Book of Infinite Wisdom*. San Francisco: Tao Publishing.

Chia, Mantak. 1983. *Awaken Healing Energy of the Tao*. Santa Fe: Aurora Press.

_____, and Maneewan Chia. 1986. *Healing Love: Cultivating Female Sexual Energy*. Huntington, NY: Healing Tao Books.

_____, and Maneevan Chia. 1996. *The Multi-Orgasmic Man*. Huntington, NY: Healing Tao Books.

_____, and Maneevan Chia. 2000. *The Multi-Orgasmic Couple: Sexual Secrets Every Couple Should Know*. San Francisco: Harper.

Chu, Valentin. 1994. *The* Yin-yang *Butterfly: Ancient Chinese Sexual Secrets for Western Lovers*. Los Angeles: J. P. Tarcher.

Cleary, Thomas. 1994. *Sex, Health, and Long Life: Manuals of Taoist Practice*. Boston: Shambala.

Comfort, Alex. 1972. *The Joy of Sex*. New York : Destiny Books.

Despeux, Catherine, and Livia Kohn. 2003. *Women in Daoism*. Cambridge, Mass.: Three Pines Press.

Douglas, Nik, and Penny Slinger. 1979. *Sexual Secrets: The Alchemy of Ecstasy*. New York: Destiny Books.

Dumas, Felice. 1997. *Passion Play*. New York: Berkeley Books.

Eliade, Mircea. 1978. *The Forge and the Crucible*. Chicago: University of Chicago Press.

Eskildsen, Stephen. 1998. *Asceticism in Early Taoist Religion*. Albany: State University of New York Press.

Girardot, Norman. 1983. *Myth and Meaning in Early Taoism*. Berkeley: University of California Press.

Jarrett, Lonny S. 1999. *Nourishing Destiny: The Inner Tradition of Chinese Medicine*. Stockbridge, Mass.: Spirit Path Press.

Liu, Xun. 2001. "To Enter the Chamber: The Ethos of Duo Practice in Ming Inner Alchemy." Paper presented at the conference on Daoist Cultivation, Vashon Island.

Lu, Kuan-yü. 1970. *Taoist Yoga: Alchemy and Immortality*. London: Rider.

Piontek, Maitreyi. 2001. *Exploring the Hidden Power of Sexuality*. New York: Samuel Weiser.

Rajneesh, Bhagwan Shree. 1971. *From Sex to Super Consciousness*. Bombay: Jeevan Jagruti Kendra.

Ruan, Fang Fu. 1991. *Sex In China: Studies in Sexology in Chinese Culture*. New York: Plenum Press.

Skar, Lowell, and Fabrizio Pregadio. 2000. "Inner Alchemy (*Neidan*)." In *Daoism Handbook*, edited by Livia Kohn, 464-97. Leiden: E. Brill.

Tortchinov, Evgeni. 1997. "The Doctrine of the Mysterious Female in Daoism." In *Everything Is According to the Way*, edited by T. R. Soidla and S. I. Shapiro. Brisbane, Australia: Bolda-Lok Publishing.

Wik, Mieke, and Stephan Wik. 2005. *Beyond Tantra: Healing through Taoist Sacred Sex*. Forres, Scotland: Findhorn Press.

Wile, Douglas. 1992. *Art of the Bedchamber: The Chinese Sexology Classics*. Albany: State University of New York Press.

Wilhelm, Richard. 1962. *The Secret of the Golden Flower*. New York: Harcourt, Brace and World.

Winn, Michael. 2001. "Daoist Alchemy as a Deep Language for Communicating with Nature." Paper presented at the conference on Daoist Cultivation, Vashon Island. www.healingdao.com/cgi-bin/articles.pl.

_____. 2002a. "The Quest for Spiritual Orgasm: Daoist and Tantric Sexuality in the West." Paper presented at the conference on Tantra and Daoism, Boston University. www.healingdao.com/cgi-bin/articles.pl.

_____, and Mantak Chia. 1984. *Taoist Secrets of Love: Cultivating Male Sexual Energy*. Santa Fe: Aurora Press.

Chapter Seven

Taiji Quan:

Forms, Visions, and Effects

BEDE BIDLACK

How wonderful is Taiji quan,
Whose movements follow nature!
Continuous like a jade bracelet,
Every movement expresses the Great Ulti-
mate.
The whole body is filled with one unbroken
qi,
Above and below are without imbalance.

Place the feet with cat steps,
Move the *qi* like coiling silk.
In movement, everything moves
In stillness, all is still.

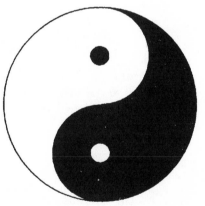

Above, the crown of the head is suspended,
And below the *qi* sinks to the elixir field.
All of this is a function of the mind,
And has nothing to do with brute force.
When full and empty are clearly distinguished,
Hard and soft follow the changing situation.
    —Li Yiyu[1]

---

[1] Li Yiyu (1832-1920) was an important Taiji quan master of the nine-
teenth century. He studied with a disciple of the founder of the Yang style
and became part of the Hao style. He also wrote extensively on the art. The
translation of the poem follows Wile 1996, 50-51.

Taiji quan (Tai Chi Chuan 太極拳), literally "Great Ultimate Boxing," in the West typically evokes ideas of groups of Chinese seniors in a park moving their hands and feet slowly and deliberately. Attracted to this exotic scene, one senses that there is a deeper meaning, a richer significance to what is happening. These people know something. What is it? What is the secret to Taiji quan that brings these people outside in all sorts of weather only to move slowly in a choreographed pattern?

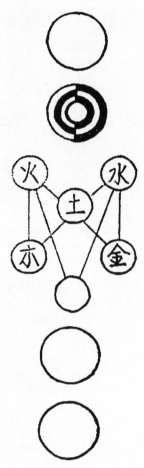

To inquire into Taiji quan in the West is to find either a dearth or a glut of schools, depending on where one lives. The metropolitan areas have the greater selection. Upon entering into a Taiji quan studio—rarely are classes offered outdoors, as in China—one notices that there are some elderly people, but there are also men and women of every age and background: doctors, lawyers, businessmen, artists, poets, social activists. What attracts such a wide variety of people to this art, peculiar to Chinese culture?

Taiji quan is a multi-faceted martial art, usually studied as a form of exercise. Some of the bene-fits of a sustained practice are good health and youthful vigor. Others include strength, grace, and martial acumen. But the secret, the mystery behind it, remains elusive. To understand Taiji quan better, the following examines its cosmo-logical background, basic principles, historical and cultural roots, as well as contemporary prac-tice and Daoist connections.

Fig. 1. The *Taiji tu*.

Cosmology

The cosmology of Taiji quan focuses on the concept of the Great Ulti-mate (Taiji 太極), a name for the universe at the time of creation, when yin and yang are present but are not yet differentiated into the five phases. Formulated first by Neo-Confucian thinkers of the Song dynasty (960-1260), the Great Ultimate is thought to arise from the Non-Ultimate (*wuji* 無極), commonly depicted as an empty circle. This represents the world before creation, at its most primordial. After evolving, the Great Ultimate, shown as interlocking patterns of black and white or yin and yang, develops the universe through the interaction of the five phases. From this basis, religious practitioners strive for a reunification with the state of creation, hoping to revert the process of evolution.

As shown in the "Taiji Diagram" in Figure 1 on the previous page, this cosmology provides the rationale for Taiji quan as a form of body cultivation, which improves health and long life and aids in the ultimate goal of a return to cosmic origins accompanied by the creation of inner harmony. In its historical roots, however, Taiji quan is also a powerful martial art, grounded traditionally in its efficacy as a fighting practice. All three aspects of the practice—cosmic, longevity, and martial—are joined, moreover, by the philosophical system of the Great Ultimate as popularized in the late Ming (1368-1644) and early Qing (1644-1911) dynasties. Tying Taiji quan to Neo-Confucian thought made it appealing to Qing literati who would otherwise be more involved in the arts of the gentleman, such as painting, calligraphy, and poetry. In this context, literati like Li Yiyu 李亦畬, who wrote the poem cited in the beginning, began to formulate philosophical and cosmological concepts of martial practice (cf. Wile 1996).

A popular text used to this end was the *Yijing* 易經 (Book of Changes), a Zhou-dynasty (ca. 1027-221 B.C.E.) divination manual which, in conjunction with its major early commentaries, also contains large portions of practical, moral advice and extensive philosophical speculations about the functioning of the universe (see Wilhelm 1950). One key focus of the text is yin-yang cosmology. "One yin, one yang, that is the Dao," says the "Great Commentary." Yin represents darkness, potentiality, the feminine, the esoteric, Earth; yang connects to light, activity, the masculine, the exoteric, Heaven. Before them, there is only the Non-Ultimate, and in their state of nascence they are called the Great Ultimate. Both the terms and the concepts are firmly rooted in the *Yijing*, and their interplay and complementary nature represent the foundation of all that exists.

One characteristic of *Yijing* and yin-yang cosmology is the idea of natural unfolding through the constancy of interactive flow. Neo-Confucian and Daoist thinkers have used this notion not only to show how the world came into being and is constantly recreated but also to create a model of human behavior on earth. Rather than attempting to manipulate circumstances to one's pleasure, they contest, it is more useful and advantageous to cooperate with circumstances and to make best use of the natural tendencies already present. This model of a balanced, ordered response in accordance with nature is also key to the understanding of Taiji quan.

As the poem by Li Yiyu notes, its movements "follow nature," are "continuous like a jade bracelet," and "express the Great Ultimate." Like yin and yang in a closely interactive, continuous, and uninhibited flow, the practitioner of Taiji quan becomes part of the an unbroken *qi* or moving energy of the cosmos, while at the same time participating in the eternal stillness of Dao underlying all. Thus the poem says: "In movement, everything moves, in stillness, all is still." Deeply rooted in and harmonious with cosmic energy, the practitioner can follow the changing situation whatever it may be.

Not only connecting to physical practice, the cosmology of Taiji quan also notes that "all is a function of the mind." Mind moves *qi*, and *qi* moves the body. Mind in its general aspect (*xin* 心) initiates the overall decision to move the *qi* and through it the body in a particular way. Mind in its particular or focused dimension as intention (*yi* 意) then effects the particulars of execution. For example, my mind decides that I want to cross the street, but my intention motivates the feet to start walking. In Taiji quan this means that the mind decides on a particular movement, such as "push," while the intention moves the *qi*, which in turn moves the hands, feet, and the rest of the body into the required position. All this happens subconsciously and instantly, the two aspects of mentation working together so closely they may almost seem inseparable (Yang 1986, 31).

As a result, advanced Taiji quan practitioners reach a state where they minimally use their physical bodies by moving their minds, which then move their *qi* and consequently their bodies. Their muscles become loose and relaxed, allowing *qi* to flow freely through the body, creating a state of health—defined in Chinese medicine as the presence of abundant, free-flowing *qi* (cf. Zheng 1985); Kaptchuk 2000; Kohn 2005). This state of health and mental focus, moreover, is the foundation not only of an extended longevity but also of spiritual attainments, a sense of oneness with the cosmos, and the realization of Daoist immortality. The cosmological roots of Taiji quan, therefore, lay the foundation for all levels of practice, from the health-oriented through the martial to the divine and spiritual.

Basic Principles

To begin the practice, adepts need to follow certain basic principles that are common to all so-called internal or soft martial arts. These stand in contrast to the external or hard-style martial arts, such as the well-known Chinese forms of Shaolin 少林 and Gongfu (Kung Fu 功夫) or the Japanese Judo 柔道, Karate 空手, and so on. The latter emphasize muscular strength (*li* 力) and require the dexterity and range of motion associated with youthful athletes. While some can practice these techniques into old age, most find that their skills deteriorate as they get older and that strength and dexterity are gradually lost.

In contrast to this, internal martial arts emphasize the springiness, or tenacity, of the muscles, tendons, and ligaments; the proper alignment of the skeletal structure; and the development of *qi*—all in the service of enhanced internal suppleness (*jin* 勁). Even though the body ages, muscles can maintain their tenacity. As a result, Taiji quan skills improve with age, and often hard-style practitioners move into Taiji quan as they get older. Hard-stylists discover the limits of their bodies and see Taiji quan as an opportunity to continue their love for the martial arts while still improving their suppleness and skill.

Whether old or young, new to the practice or transferring from hard styles, all follow several basic principles, which were conflated from ten to five by Zheng Manqing 鄭曼青 (cf. Chen 1983). The most important among them is letting go or release (*fangsong* 放送), sometimes also translated as "relax," which commonly implies that one does not use any effort at all. In contrast to this, the idea of release in Taiji quan means that one applies only the amount of effort necessary, so that one may feel relaxed but is alert and active (Cohen 1997, 98). This is the task of the mind in its different aspects: first the general mind becomes aware of tension and resolves to release it, then the intention moves to effect the release.

In this way, releasing is active. Since *qi* cannot flow through tension, letting go is an essential first step in Taiji quan (Cohen 1997, 100). It also marks a key difference to the external styles, where practitioners tighten their muscles to gain greater capacity and use a great deal of strength and external force. In Taiji quan one tightens the muscles only as much as necessary for the situation at hand and lets go of all superfluous tension. The amount of remaining tension, moreover, is so miniscule yet effective that, when coupled with the proper tech-nique, "four ounces [of suppleness] can deflect a thousand pounds [of brute force]." Students quickly learn that a shoulder that is otherwise relaxed can keep a hand elevated just as well as a shoulder that is tense with exertion.

While the principle of release most obviously applies to the body, it also works with mental and spiritual tensions. All attitudes, disposi-tions, and mental foci must be equally relaxed. That is to say, one lets go of the mind by allowing distracting thoughts to come and go with no more notice than one gives to passing clouds, creating a state of ease. However focused, this is not concentration, which implies a mind in exertion, a mind that works hard to push out distracting thoughts. Concentration of this type often leads to frustration and tension when new thoughts arise ceaselessly. The practitioner tries to push harder and exerts more effort. The relaxed mind, on the other hand, does none of this. It uses only minimal effort, enough to ignore passing thoughts.

Furthermore, to aid the body, mind, and spirit in this practice, the mind is given a home base where all or a portion of it—depending on the exercise—should rest. This point is the elixir or cinnabar field (*dantian* 丹田), located three fingers' width below the navel and three fingers' width inside the body. As Li's poem notes, "below the *qi* sinks to the elixir field; all of this is a function of the mind." Similarly, Zheng Manqing says: "Sink the *qi* to the elixir field; move the *qi* with the mind and the body with the *qi*" (Zheng 1985, 13). As the mind sinks into the abdomen, the *qi* follows, and this in turn causes the body to respond. The response is diaphragmatic breathing. Breathing deeply into the abdomen increases lung capacity and oxygenation of the body. It enhances *qi* and affords greater relaxation and focus, which in turn make the practice of release easier. Release, abdominal breathing, and a mental focus on the elixir field are thus mutually supportive. With body and mind in this open state, one is free to prac-tice with a sense of ease, regardless of success and failure. Conse-quently the spirit is free of tension.

Having found a firm base in release or letting go one can move on to the next principle of practice: verticality. On the surface, verticality means keeping the body upright; on a deeper level it means to main-tain a seamless, energetic connection in the body from the top of the head to the soles of the feet. Although everybody is naturally endowed with this *qi*-connection, people commonly sever it by creating tension in the lower back at a point called Gate of Life (*mingmen* 命門), located on the lumbar spine at about the level of the kidneys. Tension here blocks the *qi* and leaves the body divided in two pieces: the upper torso and the lower body. Verticality thus means opening this area so that one can perform each movement with the entire body and can allow the movement to reach easily from feet to head and head to feet. As the *Taiji quan shiyong fa* 太極拳使用法 (Applications of Taiji Quan), an early text citing a revelation from Zhang Sanfeng, says:

> The root is in the feet; the *qi* issues up through the legs. It is controlled by the waist and is expressed in the hands and fingers. From the feet to the legs to the waist should be one complete flow of *qi*. (Wile 1983, 102)

Different styles have different ways of opening the lower back. For example, the masters of the Wu style teach practitioners to lean the upper body slightly forward and to straighten the lower back; Yang style masters, on the other hand, advise to roll under the tail bone in a pelvic tilt.

Closely related to verticality, third, is the principle of the centrality of the body's middle, expressed in the texts as "the waist is the commander." Centrality here means that the hands do not move unless the waist is moving. The waist, like the fulcrum of a clock, is the central, coordinating device for all moves. Even though different parts of the body, like the different hands of a clock, move at different speeds, the waist coordinates them all so that they operate as one unit. If the principle of verticality allows practitioners to move as one body, the principle of centrality makes this happen.

Once verticality and centrality are found, one can move on to do the first actual move, following the next principle, which is called "empty stepping" or "stepping like a cat." This is a very concrete principle. Imagine a cat stalking prey. Notice how the cat lifts one paw cleanly from the ground, carefully places it down, then puts its weight on it. Moving like this, Taiji quan practitioners gain the balance and sure-footedness that attracts many people to the art. In the beginning, students often think it means that the entire weight should always be on one leg; however, this is only a training technique for empty stepping. Rarely does one keep all of the weight on one leg for very long. Empty stepping means that there is always the *potential* for moving into the other leg while emptying the standing leg (cf. Sim and Gaffney 2001).

To do empty stepping correctly, step out and place the foot down gently, then slowly push into it so that the weight fills the leg gradually from the foot up. Do not fall into the leg, filling it from the top down as most people do when walking—having already lost the principle of verticality. As they walk, people tend to move their weight forward expecting that their foot will land on solid ground. When that happens, their weight goes into the foot from the top down. If it does not land properly—if there is a blockage or a hole—their weight is already in forward motion and they stumble or trip. Accordingly, the more Taiji quan practitioners nurture empty stepping the less they stumble or trip, even in daily life.

The last major principle of Taiji quan practice concerns the arms and hands. Called "fair lady's wrist," it requires that the wrists be kept completely relaxed, allowing the *qi* to flow to the hands and, most importantly, to the point in the center of the palms. Known as Labor Palace (*laogong* 勞宮), this point is a major passageway of *qi* in and out of the body. External *qi* healers use it to infuse energy into patients; other *qi* practitioners activate it to keep their *qi* flow steady. In Taiji quan and other martial arts it is important as the point that makes most frequent contact with others, be they partners or opponents. Any tension in the wrist that causes the *qi* to be blocked makes it impossible to release it through the palms and cancels out any effort at striking or pushing, leaving the practitioner striving in vain.

Forms in History

Taiji quan first developed in the seventeenth century in the village of a family named Chen in Wenxian County, Henan (Sim and Gaffney 2001, 1). Chen Wangting 陳王廷, a military officer under the Ming, was released from service as the Manchus conquered China and established the Qing dynasty in the 1640s. He returned home and developed a martial work-out that helped to keep him and his village healthy and able to defend against marauding troops.[2] He studied the *Quanshu* 拳書 (Book of Boxing) by the Ming general Qi Jiguang 戚繼光 and created the first five Taiji quan forms, not only using martial training but also integrating healing exercises (Daoyin) and Neo-Confucian cosmology. His method came to be known as Chen style Taiji quan. It is characterized by its explosive style that involves stomping, leaping, and even yelling. A slow, smooth movement can

---

[2] See Sim and Gaffney 2001, 1; Kohn 2005, 195; Wile 1983, ii; Despeux 1981, 22.

quickly end in a snapping punch, while the practitioner lets out a loud *he*!

More popular today is Yang style practice, made famous by Yang Lu-chan 楊露禪 (1799-1872). He was a disciple of Chen Zhangxing 陳長興 (1771-1853), a descendant of the original founder. Various stories tell how Yang found his way into Chen discipleship. According to one, Yang had heard of the Chens' renown as martial artists and wanted to study with them, but the family did not teach its art to outsiders. As a result, Yang took to spying on their in-family instruction through a window. He practiced what he saw and became so adept that the Chens eventually accepted him as a disciple. Quickly rising to superior expertise, Yang left the village to win matches wherever he went. By the time he made his way to Beijing, he was called "Yang the Invincible." Invited to teach the elite military banner men of the Manchu-Qing dynasty, he could not refuse, but being a Han Chinese and Ming loyalist, he did not wish them to have the full power of his art (Wile 1983iiiff.). Instead, he taught them a modified form, which later came to be called the public as opposed to the original, esoteric or "secretly transmitted" (*michuan* 秘傳) style (cf. Rodell 2003).

The public and esoteric forms differ mainly in that the public form requires most of the weight being placed in the front leg, while the esoteric style emphasizes the rear leg (Rodell 2003, 35ff.). Also, taking only about twenty-five minutes versus over an hour for the esoteric pattern, the public form is shorter and less intricate. When compared to the older Chen style, according to some, Yang-family Taiji quan is more martial (Sim and Gaffney 200123), but most agree that its movements, lacking any explosions, are more uniform in pace and smoother than those of the Chen style.

Both versions of Yang style practice were transmitted by Yang Lu-chan to his son Yang Jianhou 楊健侯 (1839-1917), who passed the public form on to his son Yang Chenfu 楊澄甫 (1883-1936). Yang Chenfu taught it to the non-family practitioner Zhang Qinlin 張欽霖 (1887-1976), who also learned the esoteric style from Yang Jianhou. While Yang focused on the public form, Zhang became the key expo-nent of the esoteric version. The public form, moreover, made it into the United States when Yang Chenfu's charismatic student Zheng Manqing 鄭曼青 (1900-1975) arrived in New York in the 1970s. The esoteric form reached Taiwan with Zhang's student Wang Yannian (王延年, b. 1914), a military officer who left the mainland in 1949. Af-ter receiving permission from Zhang to teach the form to a wider audience, he made it available to thousands of students and has since created a considerable following in the West (cf. Wang 1988).

The third major style of Taiji quan is Wu style. It goes back to the original founder of the Yang style who also taught a Manchurian bodyguard by the name of Wu Quanyou 吳全佑 (1834-1902). His son Wu Jianquan 吳監泉 (1870-1942) in due course popularized the form developed by his father and made it into the Wu style known today. It is characterized by a large waist rotation, narrow stance, and a slanted back from the rear foot to the top of the head (Sim and Gaffney 2001, 23).

A yet different style is called Hao. It originated with another prominent student of Yang Luchan called Wu Yuxiang 武禹襄 (ca. 1812-1880). However, Wu not only worked with Yang but also studied under a member of the Chen family and ended up combining elements of the two styles. His pattern is known as Hao because of its main representative Hao Weizhan 郝爲楨 (1849-1920), a student of Wu's nephew Li Yiyu (1832-1920). Because Li was a rather famous figure in his own right, this style is sometimes also called Li style (Sim and Gaffney 2001, 24). The form is characterized by high and compact stances, handwork that never crosses the body, and an emphasis on rising and falling, opening and closing. It is the least known in the West today (Sim and Gaffney 2001, 25).

Despite this fact, the Hao lineage is responsible for most written works on Taiji quan before the twentieth century, superseded later by numerous books and articles issuing from members of the Yang family, especially attributed to Yang Chenfu. Considered as "Taiji quan classics," these texts describe forms, principles, practice types, and philosophical perspectives (see Wile 1996; 2003; Davis 2004).

Practice Variations

All these major schools and forms of Taiji quan encourage students to practice in a variety of ways. Most commonly, they begin training in solo movements, incorporating the five principles and learning the cosmological and spiritual implications of the art. Solo practice is a valuable foundation and, like any challenging art or skill, requires time and perseverance to learn. Practitioners have to replace old physical habits with new ones, tirelessly repeating movements until they become completely natural. Unless they gain these new ways of moving and being in the body, their movements remain within the old realm of muscular strength, aggressive thinking, and lack of balance and alignment. Time, regular practice, and abundant patience are thus key ingredients to success in Taiji quan.

Once they have mastered the solo form, students may hone their skills by practicing with a partner in various forms of pushing hands or sparring. They apply their newly learned techniques to multiple situations that challenge their stance, mental focus, and movements. Learning greater subtlety in this partner-based application, they improve their solo form and become advanced practitioners. The same also holds true for weapons practice, which can involve swords, poles, fans, or other instruments. Practitioners learn to project their *qi* into the weapon and to increase their precision and fluidity of movement. All three practice variations are essential to the complete understanding of Taiji quan.

SOLO PRACTICE. Beginners start by practicing the solo form, a combination of carefully choreographed movements with a fixed beginning and end. To begin, practitioners stand with their feet together and their hands loose by their sides, with the head erect and the eyes open. They breathe deeply into the abdomen and clear outside thoughts from their minds to become completely present. The form ends with practitioners in the same posture, after a more or less complex sequence of movements and postures that involve focused breathing, alternating the weight in the feet, and striking or blocking with the hands. The movements are slow, continuous, and purposeful; they are at all times coordinated with the breath. Length varies, depending on the form and the speed of practice (see Fig. 2).

In addition to the four major styles, Taiji quan has many forms which vary according to length (long, short), transmission (public, esoteric), and number of moves (37, 49, or 108). Any master may create a new variation or choose to emphasize different aspects of the practice. However, the particular styles have their clear overall characteristics, and solo practice in general has a number of important benefits for health and personality. Practitioners gain greater mental acuity, improved muscle tone, flexibility, cardiovascular health, and blood circulation. They also experience a decrease in stress and tension and an increase in overall mental and physical well-being. From the point of view of Chinese medicine, practitioners gain a greater abundance of *qi* as well as a better balance and *qi*-flow throughout mind, body and spirit (Wang 2004; Smalheiser 2004).

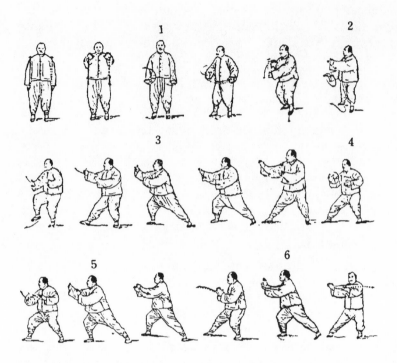

Fig. 2: A sequence of Taiji quan

ENGAGING THE PARTNER. Many schools also require practitioners to train with a partner. The word for partner is *duifang* 對方, which literally means "facing direction" and by extension indicates the "opposite." The term emphasizes the joined and interdependent nature of the two partners engaged in the exercise. They are not strictly speaking opponents or attackers, terms that evoke mental attitudes of separateness, competition, and fear. All these are counterproductive to Taiji quan, which aims to cultivate perception, connection, and coordinated movement.

Since they must perform in close contact, working with a partner challenges practitioners. It provides a vastly different experience from solo practice, where one is free to move at one's own pace and can make mistakes without immediate feedback. Another benefit of partner practice is that adepts appreciate the martial application of the solo form. It enhances the work in the various applications and leads to the ability to execute all moves easily and without inhibition or uncertainty. Certain moves that seemed senseless or vague before come into clearer focus. For example, someone may not have been completely clear how the movement "push" worked. Now, by actually pushing against another person, the practitioner will learn how "push" feels and how the partner responds. Returning to solo practice, this person may attempt to replicate that feeling, thereby correcting any errors, such as leaning too much into one or the other direction.

Partner practice comes in three major forms: roll back, push hands, and free hands. Roll back (*dalu* 大履) is similar to solo practice in that it is choreographed, has a formal beginning and end, and comes with several variations. However, it tends to be shorter and consists of fewer movements than the solo form. Its purpose is to develop livelier stepping with proper distancing from the partner.

In contrast to roll back, where variation is limited and the movements are predictable, the practice of push hands (*tuishou* 推手) is unpredictable and largely unrestrained by choreography. An exercise designed to hone martial skills of perception and response, push hands may involve no stepping, limited and linear stepping, or free stepping. These three are also called fixed step, restricted step, and moving step. The aim of the practice is to upset the partner's root (i.e., their connection with the floor) and to explore greater subtleties in the mutual exchange.

While push hands focuses on working with the arms and hands and does not include kicks or strikes, the third form of partner practice includes everything. Known as free hands (*sanshou* 散手), it has only one rule, and that is the rule of common sense. In this respect it is different from sparring, which has specific rules and a detailed point system. Before they engage in free hands, students of Taiji quan should have practiced with teachers and classmates for at least a year and should have developed strong ties of trust and friendship. Mutual respect, practical experience, and self-control will prevent them from executing aggressive moves that might endanger their partner. Anyone showing signs of being overly aggressive will probably not be invited to the free hand class or have difficulty finding practice partners. Also, aggressive people rarely have the patience to take the year or so to learn the solo form and basic push hands, which are prerequisites for free hands practice.

Free hands training serves to develop practitioners' full range of Taiji quan dynamics. It allows them to experiment with different kinds of attacks, angles, paces, kicks, and even grappling (cf. Yang 1995). It represents the highest level of physical training and opens practitioners to the full range of possibilities: what they can do, what they can expect, and how they can fail. Failure is as good a teacher as success. Like push hands, it informs the form, and the form gives the practitioner different movements to try. Partner work and solo practice are thus two sides of the same coin. As Zheng Manqing puts it:

> Some skeptics say that [Taiji quan] has no practical function and cast it aside; some hold that it serves only health and do not look beyond this. They do not understand that the principles and applications of this martial art are as inseparable as form and shadow. If one studies, but cannot put his knowledge to practice, then what he has gained from the principles will be false. (Zheng 1985, 6)

WEAPONS TRAINING. Taiji quan training is not complete without weapons practice. Like empty-handed boxing (quan 拳), it comes in solo and various partner forms and has the same basic benefits, such as enhanced qi, open joints, increased agility, better balance, and heightened mental focus. In addition, the increased challenge of handling a weapon brings out these benefits even more.

For example, in the sword training known as Taiji jian 太極檢 practitioners work with a straight, double-bladed sword. Doing so, they not only have a difference in weight and energy in one hand, but they can also use the sword as an object to push against and gain the opportunity to practice the release of *qi* from the hand into the sword. Practicing with a weapon increases the precision of the moves. Instead of working with the hand and its diameter of four inches targeting objects of roughly the same size, they now use the tip of the sword to aim at targets only about an inch in diameter. Beyond demanding heightened focus and precision, this also makes mistakes easier to notice and increases awareness of possible shortcomings in Taiji quan practice. If the tip of the sword wavers or moves past the intended target, it is likely that the same error occurs in the practitioner's empty-handed form. The sword thus becomes a magnifying glass for practice deficiencies.

The same also holds true for practice with the spear or pole (*gan* 杆), typically a wooden stick eight to twelve feet long. However, the pole is much heavier than the sword and thus more difficult to wield. The pole is maneuvered at the end, not in the middle, with techniques usable with a spear, such as parry, pierce, and block. For this reason, the names are interchangeable. Its weight and momentum require adepts to develop excellent balance, superior openness, and good inner-body connection. They must resist the temptation to use muscular strength, instead relying on the suppleness and internal tenacity developed in basic practice.

Sword and spear with their moderate and heavy weight are the two most common weapons in Taiji quan. But practitioners also use the fan (*fengshan* 風扇), an extremely light weapon, and the saber (*dao* 刀), a single, curved-bladed sword. Fan movements are quick and light, as the practitioner opens and closes the fan. Once made of metal and quite sturdy, fans could be used like clubs when closed and served to conceal an approaching strike or distract an opponent when open. Saber practitioners use large round movements, since the shape of the saber is conducive for slicing, rather than poking or chopping, like the straight sword. In addition, its single blade prevents the practitioner from cutting in two directions, but the dull edge allows for movements that would be unwise for a double bladed sword, such as swinging the blade over one's head or supporting the blade with the free hand against the dull side.

Other instruments are less martial and involve the cultivation of internal energy. They are the ball and the ruler, a stick used for strengthening the joints (Yang 1986, 18-19; Sim and Gaffney 2001, 143-48). These instruments are used in advanced practice to develop energetic power in a way that would harm a partner if one were to use them on another person. Taiji stick (*bang* 棒) is an exercise for increasing strength and flexibility in the wrists, hands, elbows, and shoulders for grappling movements (*qinna* 擒拿). The stick is roughly ten inches in length and two inches thick. Using the whole body in circular movements, the practitioner twists the stick to imitate the locks and counter movements of grappling. One concentrates on developing flexibility and twisting strength, as well as the ability to close the chest and waist.

All these different forms of Taiji quan are potent and helpful for healing and serve to prepare practitioners for spiritual attainments and to give them the basic guidelines for the more advanced path. They are subtle and helpful and serve to create a good foundation for the Daoist quest of transcendence and immortality.

The Daoist Connection

Daoists did not invent Taiji quan nor was it traditionally a major form of Daoist cultivation. The connection was established in the mid-Qing dynasty when Zhang Sanfeng 張三丰, a rather elusive Daoist of the early Ming and immortal associated with Mount Wudang 武當山 in Hunan, manifested during a séance and dictated his spiritual autobiography, claiming excellence in martial practice and the creation of several self-cultivation forms.[3] Picking up on this potent revelation, Taiji quan followers created a story that linked Yang Luchan to the divine origin of the art. According to this tale, the elder Chen gave Yang the methods transmitted by Zhang Sanfeng, which Yang pursued by journeying to Mount Wudang where he studied Daoist meditation and the soft aspects of the martial arts (Wile 1983, vii).

Since then, Zhang Sanfeng has been the major saint of Taiji quan, as is evidenced by the Zhang Sanfeng Festival, held in Pennsylvania in early June every year (see www.americansocietyofinternalarts.org), where Taiji quan and Qigong practitioners exchange workshops and techniques. Similarly, Mount Wudang in China has become an important center of Daoist martial arts, modeling its organization and practice after the successful Shaolin Temple 少林寺, the headquarters of Buddhist martial practice located at the foot of Mount Song 嵩山 near Luoyang.

Discovered by the Hong Kong film industry in the 1980s as a source of phenomenal stuntmen and fighters, the Shaolin temple complex has become a martial Disneyland, with tourists and students flocking to it by the thousands and new construction booming every year. Daoists of Mount Wudang have similarly succeeded in creating a popular image of the Daoist monk as martial savant and actively promote the image of Taiji quan as Daoist practice. In fact, Wudang style practitioners claim that their form is at the root of all internal martial arts and that it contains all different styles.[4] As a result, a similar boom as at Shaolin is beginning on Mount Wudang, and other Daoist centers are eager to market their own forms. They benefit from the publicity, the income that tourists and students provide, as well as from the sale of books and tapes that feature their monks. Inter-monastery

---

[3] On Zhang Sanfeng and his legends, see Seidel 1970; Wong 1982; DeBruyn 2000. On the importance of Mount Wudang and its central deity, the Dark Warrior, see Lagerwey 1992.

[4] Louis Komjathy, personal communication, June 2005.

competitions are the latest fad in this exceptional Daoist boom of Taiji quan (see Fig. 3).

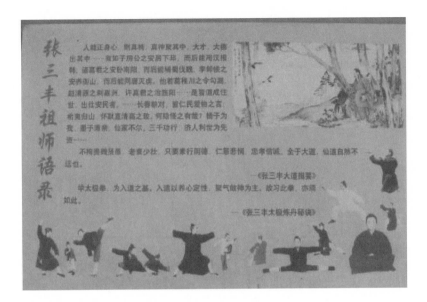

Fig. 3. Poster at the White Cloud Monastery showing Taiji quan moves and sayings by Zhang Sanfeng.

To justify the connection, Daoists both of the Qing dynasty and today have argued that Taiji quan and Daoism share basic cosmological concepts such as yin and yang and that the practice in many ways benefits religious and spiritual training. Cited most frequently in this context is the cosmic dimension expressed through the *Taiji tu* diagram (Fig. 1 above) which teaches an experience of harmony with Heaven and Earth and the reversion of particularity back to the formlessness before creation through the return to a spontaneous, child-like existence both in body and mind.

Creation and reversion are both expressed in Taiji quan forms. Practitioners begin by standing motionless and being free of thought, then move in symbolic separation of yin and yang, lifting the hands as yang energy rises to create Heaven and lowering them as yin energy sinks to create Earth. Like the creation of the myriad beings, the movements transform from posture to posture without pause. In the end, the hands drop and the feet come together. Practitioners find stillness and return to formlessness.

Philosophical and cosmological reflection upon Taiji quan is very rich. Shared by Daoists and Neo-Confucians alike, it focuses on the unfolding of Dao into the two forces of yin and yang and on the interaction of Heaven, Earth, and Humanity. As Yang Chenfu says:

> If one can understand the principle of the reversal of yin and yang, then we can begin to discuss the Dao. When one understands the Dao and can maintain this without lapse, then we can begin to discuss humanity. When one can magnify the Dao by means of humanity, and know that the Dao is not apart from it, then we can begin to discuss the unity of Heaven and Earth.
>
> Heaven is above and Earth below; humanity occupies the center. If one can explore the Heavens and examine the Earth . . . then we can speak of [the cosmos as] the macrocosmic Heaven and Earth and humanity as the microcosmic Heaven and Earth.
>
> Extend your knowledge and investigate the world through the wisdom and abilities of Heaven and Earth. This, then, may be called innate human wisdom and skill. If one's thoughts never depart from the truth, they will have a powerful effect. If one's great *qi* is properly nourished and not damaged, it will endure forever. This is what we mean by the human body comprising a Heaven and Earth in miniature.
>
> Heaven is one's nature and Earth one's life. The light and sensitive in human beings is the spirit. If the spirit is not pure, how can one fulfill the role of third partner along with Heaven and Earth? What is the meaning of existence if one does not fulfill one's nature, cultivate life, expand the spirit, and evolve positively? (Wile 1983, 136)

Joining Heaven and Earth as a fully conscious third partner, human beings practicing Taiji quan can pursue the Daoist ideal of spontaneity (*ziran* 自然), found already in the *Daode jing* as the highest factor in the universe:

> The king patterns himself on Earth,
> Earth patterns itself on Heaven,
> Heaven patterns itself on the Dao.
> And the Dao patterns itself on spontaneity. (ch. 25)

Similarly, the *Zhuangzi* describes the Daoist ideal of the skilled craftsman who can fully follow the spontaneous workings of nature and the world. In one story, Wheelwright Slab tells Duke Huan about the method for finding Dao:

> Your servant looks at it from the point of view of his own business. When I chisel a wheel, if I hit too softly, it slips and won't bite. If I hit too hard, it jams and won't move. Neither too soft nor too hard—I get it in my hand and respond with my mind. But my mouth cannot put it into words. There is an art to it. But your servant can't show it to his own son, and he can't get it from me. I've done it this way seventy years and am growing old chiseling wheels. (Ivanhoe and Van Norden 2003)

In this vision, Dao is found by way of concrete practice and experience. Wheelwright Slab "cannot put it into words." There are no rules to follow, no signposts or guidelines: "There is an art to it." The craftsman must respond to Dao, manifest in the wheel he is carving: "Neither too soft nor too hard: I get it in my hand and respond with my mind." In this way he learns over the course of sustained practice—"I've done it this way seventy years"—to reverse the process of socialization in order to move in a more spontaneous manner with the Dao.

The same holds true for the art of Taiji quan. Through sustained practice, one reverts to the spontaneous mental state of childhood, without the clutter of the socialized mind: the mind of limits, definitions, rules, and mores. As Dao is in the craftsman's wheel, so it also manifests itself in practitioners during solo practice and in the other during partner work. Over time one learns to move with them and thus to move with the Dao (Bidlack Forthcoming).

This awareness of the other and the flow of communal movement also add a sociological dimension to the practice. Taiji quan requires practitioners to concentrate not only within themselves but also outside, thus enhancing awareness of nature and group cohesion. Even in solo practice, often undertaken in a group, practitioners must always be aware of their position and the position of the others, knowing exactly where they are and how fast they move. In this way members of the group interact with each other even when practicing the solo form. Success comes with yielding and passivity, acting only when the time is right. If one moves either too fast or too slowly, one causes disharmony that can be felt by the entire group. Even worse, if members assert themselves, group cohesion is lost and the practice area falls into chaos.

Partner practice demands an even greater susceptibility to the moves and intentions of others. Here every move and mental flicker gives rise to an immediate parry and reaction. But one does not need an actual partner to develop this skill. Even when alone, one can visualize the partner, allowing the mind to focus on a specific target at a specific distance, and thus learn to "follow the changing situation" (Yang 1986, 24; Sim and Gffney 2001,75). As adepts in their practice are always in relationship with others and the cosmos, both mentally and spiritually, Taiji quan as a Daoist art serves the internal harmony of the community by heightening group awareness and cultivating group activity. It eases the tensions that are bound to arise when people live together in a compound over prolonged periods.

Aside from all these potent reasons why Taiji quan is a valid and popular Daoist practice today, it has also well-documented health benefits. Even in medieval times good health was considered a basic prerequisite for advanced Daoist practice, and today it is the condition for first steps in inner alchemy. As Taiji quan encourages the balanced, uninhibited flow of *qi*, it helps to restore and maintain good health. On this basis, adepts can then pursue the more advanced practice of Daoist alchemy with its goal of returning to the Dao through refining *qi*.

The entire process is centered on the body. It must not be diseased due to imbalanced or wayward *qi*, which cannot be transformed into purified *qi*. Refining *qi* into purified *qi* is the first step before one can begin to refine essence (*jing* 精)—semen for men and menstrual blood for women—into *qi* that can then be transformed into the spiritual dimension of *shen*. This advanced refinement occurs through mental effort in meditation, and again Taiji quan as a moving meditation is a good way of preparation. It trains the mind to focus and to release intruding thoughts, matching the stillness and immobility of seated practice, commonly called "sitting in oblivion" (*zuowang* 坐忘; see Kohn 1987). Using the body as an aid to meditation, the practitioner learns to enjoy mental clarity and gets ready for higher spiritual attainments.

The enhancement of health in monastic practitioners also has also a practical effect. Giving community members the responsibility for personal fitness and encouraging them to participate in a daily exercise regimen frees the monastery of the burden of excessive health care costs. To allow time for spiritual practices and liturgical services, monasteries keep worldly matters to a minimum, such as maintaining buildings and grounds, housing guests, and obtaining food and fuel. All of these items require money, which is scarce because Chinese monastics only receive minimum stipends from the state and do not earn large sums through ritual and other services. Avoiding sickness with daily Taiji quan helps to reduce expenses and thus benefits the institution as a whole.

In addition to these reasons for the practice of Taiji quan by ordained Daoists, some lay Daoist sects use Taiji quan as a window through which to judge the character of prospective members. Such sects are secretive about their practices and do not share them lightly with others. Taiji quan can reveal the aptitude of a student to a teacher. If students are sloppy and lazy in their Taiji quan practice, it is likely that they will also be slothful in their Daoist practice and are therefore not ready for more intense or advanced training. However, if they demonstrate good determination and work ethic in their Taiji quan practice, they are likely to succeed and are allowed to approach the teacher to request acceptance as a Daoist student.[5]

Conclusion

What is the secret of Taiji quan? Its secret lies in its comprehensive and surprising character. It is both martial technique and meditative art, regimen for health and discipline for self-cultivation, singular and interactive, secular and Daoist, mythical and historical. It is not a single activity of slow movements but a broad collection of exercises and techniques. It is a martial art founded by warriors of impeccable skill. Not born of Daoism, it was absorbed into it.

Taiji quan continues to surprise and challenge practitioners of all ages and backgrounds. It is these surprises along the road of self-cultivation that draw practitioners to practice day after day. The more martial techniques attract youths searching an outlet for their vigorous energy, while the meditative aspects retain and sustain the practitioner through old age.

These attributes are no secret, but the variety of spiritual and physical exercises available to the modern Western practitioner are so great and the competition for being heard so aggressive that some may miss the opportunity for discovering Taiji quan due to the siren

---

[5] Interview with Wang Yannian by Bede Bidlack, Scott Rodell, and Meilu Rodell, March 2005.

song of other exercises, meditations, or mind-body classes. In addition, students see only the solo, empty-handed form and think that this is all. As a result, they may limit their practice to this form rather than continuing on to other forms, partner and weapons practice. They may find limited solo practice boring and unrewarding.

Taking this phenomenon into account, some adepts are even forecasting the demise of Taiji quan (Yang 1986, 18; Rodell 2003, xiii). Although the complete death of the art is unlikely—especially given the fact that is has risen to be a competitive sport and occupies a place in the Beijing Olympics of 2008—it is clear that Taiji quan has changed over the centuries and continues to change. Once studied as a martial practice, it has become an efficacious method for relaxation and good health for large numbers of people. Sports enthusiasts use it to compete for greater glory, while Daoists embrace it to lay the foundation of spiritual attainment. Some even claim that it is an immortality technique which by itself will lead to transcendence. With this broad a spectrum of venues, Taiji quan will endure, but it may not be anything Chen Wangting, Yang Luchan, or the other founders would still recognize.

Bibliography

Bidlack, Bede. forthcoming. "Living on the Threshold." In *Believer's Notes*, edited by Arvind Sharma. New York: Penguin.

Chen, Weiming. 1983. "Oral Instructions from Yang Chenfu." In *Tai Chi Touchstones: Yang Family Secret Transmissions*, compiled and edited by Douglas Wile, 9-14. Brooklyn, NY: Sweet Ch'i Press.

Cohen, Kenneth. 1997. *The Way of Qi Gong.* New York: Ballantine.

Davis, Barbara. 2004. *The Taiji quan Classics: An Annotated Translation.* Berkeley: North Atlantic Books.

DeBruyn, Pierre-Henry. 2000. "Daoism in the Ming (1368-1644)." In *Daoism Handbook*, edited by Livia Kohn, 594-622. Leiden: E. Brill.

Despeux, Catherine. 1981. *Taiji Quan: Art Martial, Technique De Long Vie.* Paris: Guy Trédaniel.

Ivanhoe, Philip and Van Norden, Bryan W. 2003. *Readings in Classical Chinese Philosophy*. Indianapolis: Hackett Publishing Company.

Kaptchuk, Ted. 2000. *The Web That Has No Weaver: Understanding Chinese Medicine*. New York: Contemporary Books.

Kohn, Livia. 1987. *Seven Steps to the Tao: Sima Chengzhen's Zuowanglun*. St.Augustin/Nettetal: Monumenta Serica Monograph XX.

_____. 2005. *Health and Long Life: The Chinese Way*. Cambridge, Mass.: Three Pines Press.

Lagerwey, John. 1992. "The Pilgrimage to Wu-tang Shan." In *Pilgrims and Sacred Sites in China*, edited by Susan Naquin and Chün-fang Yü, 293-332. Berkeley: University of California Press.

Rodell, Scott M. 2003. *Chinese Swordsmanship: The Yang Family Taiji jian Tradition*. Annondale: Seven Stars Books.

Seidel, Anna. 1970. "A Taoist Immortal of the Ming Dynasty: Chang San-feng." *Self and Society in Ming Thought*, edited by Wm. Th. DeBary, 483-531. New York: Columbia University Press.

Sim, Davidine Siaw-Voon, and David Gaffney. 2001. *Chen Style Taijiquan: The Source of Taiji Boxing*. Berkley: North Atlantic Books.

Smalheiser, Marvin. 2004. "Using Science to Study Qigong, T'ai Chi." *T'ai Chi Magazine* 28: 14-20.

Wang, Chechen, et. al. 2004 "The Effect of Tai Chi on Health Outcomes in Patients with Chronic Conditions: A Systematic Review." *Archives of Internal Medicine* 164: 493-501.

Wang, Yannian. 1988. *Yangjia Michuan Taiji Quan: Illustrated and Explained*. Translated by Julia Fairchild. Taipei: Grand Hotel T'ai Chi Ch'uan Association.

Wile, Douglas. 1983. *T'ai Chi Touchstones: Yang Family Secret Transmissions*. New York: Sweet Ch'i Press.

_____. 1996. *Lost T'ai-Chi Classics From the Late Ch'ing Dynasty*. Albany: State University of New York.

Wilhelm, Richard. 1950. *The I Ching or Book of Changes*. Princeton: Princeton University Press, Bollingen Series XIX.

Wong, Shiu Hon. 1982. *Investigations into the Authenticity of the Chang San-feng ch'uan-chi.* Canberra: Australian National University Press.

Yang, Jwing-ming. 1986. *Tai Chi Theory and Martial Power: Advanced Yang Style.* Jamaica Plain, Mass.: YMAA Publications.

_____. 1995. *Comprehensive Applications of Shaolin Chin Na: The Practical Defense of Chinese Seizing Arts for All Styles, 2nd Edition.* Jamaica Plain, Mass.: YMAA Publications.

Zheng, Manqing. 1985. "Author's Preface to The New Methods of Self-Study for T'ai- Chi Ch'uan." In *Cheng Man-Ch'ing's Advanced T'ai-Chi Form Instructions*, edited by Douglas Wile, 6-33. New York: Sweet Ch'i Press.

Chapter Eight

Qigong in America[*]

LOUIS KOMJATHY

Qigong 氣功 (Ch'i-kung) most basically refers to exercises (*gong*) that involve the circulation of *qi*, a term which may refer to physical breath and a more subtle pneuma, vapor, or vital energy. In a wider cultural context, Qigong is a modern Chinese health and longevity movement with its own particular history. Only emerging in the early twentieth century and coming to prominence from the 1950s onwards, it developed as a Chinese nativist response to the challenges of a Western scientific paradigm, modernization, and colonialism. [1] Originally a syncretic and secularist phenomenon, in recent years it has come to lay more spiritual claims and has made inroads in religious organizations, both in China and the West.

---

[*] I am grateful to Livia Kohn for her helpful comments on the present article. In addition, Elijah Siegler and David Palmer provided guidance as well as made their publications available. Mark Johnson, Michael Rinaldini, Kate Townsend, Michael Winn, and other members of the American Qigong community also provided important information.

[1] In her study of modern millennial movements, Catherine Wessinger provides the following definition: "A *nativist millennial movement* consists of individuals who feel oppressed by a foreign colonizing government, believing that the government is removing the natives [*sic*] from their land and eradicating their traditional way of life" (2000, 159). If one accepts that such forms of colonization and oppression may also occur in mental spaces, and that the "foreign government" may be ideological as well as ethnic, then Qigong may be understood as an indigenous Chinese response to the ideological challenge of Communism with its secularist and materialistic worldview. That is, Communism, especially as implemented by Mao Zedong, represented a challenge to traditional Chinese culture, which culminated in the Cultural Revolution.

Qigong incorporates facets of traditional Chinese cosmological theories (yin-yang, five phases, etc.), Chinese medicine, long life pursuits, healing exercises, Daoist and Buddhist aspects, as well as Western medical and scientific paradigms. Its history resembles that of Traditional Chinese Medicine (TCM), the modern form of Chinese healing systematized by the Communist government under the influence of Western biomedicine. Like TCM, Taiji quan and Fengshui, Qigong is not Daoist in origin or essence. On the most general level, Qigong emphasizes personal health and well-being, and one could argue that this is one defining characteristic that stands in contrast to the historical contours of the Daoist tradition (see Cohen 1997; Kohn 2000; Palmer 2005; 2006).

Following the Communist revolution that resulted in the founding of the People's Republic of China in 1949 and the unleashing of the Cultural Revolution (1966-1976), Qigong spread throughout the world and is now a transnational movement. In America, Chinese immigrants first introduced it in the 1950s, with a sharp increase in practitioners when immigration laws were liberalized in 1965. The first publication solely dedicated to Qigong appeared in 1973. This period was followed by a second generation of teachers, mostly Euro-Americans who studied under Chinese immigrants or traveled to China or Taiwan for their training.

Today there are as many Qigong forms as there are Qigong teachers and organizations. As in China, Qigong in America as much as in Europe, Japan, and elsewhere is primarily a health and fitness movement that is increasingly picked up by quasi-religious groups and used for more spiritual purposes. It has become widespread mainly because of its health-enhancement and healing properties, and in the West has joined the alternative spirituality and complementary health care movements. Its popularity is thus the result of complex historical and cultural factors, including mainland Chinese politics, American immigration rules, as well as the American counter-culture, the New Age movement, and the increasing dissatisfaction with conventional health care.

Categories of Qigong

Like any large-scale cultural development, Qigong is complex and multidimensional. Four major categories may be identified: martial, medical, Buddhist, and Daoist (Miura 1989, 341-53; Liang and Wu 1997; Reid 1998, 43-63). They are somewhat problematic, since many Qigong systems are syncretic and innovative, often intentionally combining aspects from different Chinese traditions as well as utilizing the rhetoric of tradition and lineage to generate increased cultural capital. One must also distinguish emic (insider) accounts, which are often mythological ("This form originated with Hua Tuo;" "Qigong is over 5,000 years old"), from a historically nuanced understanding of the actual origins of and motivations behind such constructions (see Kohn 2001; Miller 2003).

Martial Qigong is usually associated with martial arts, Gongfu, and the so-called internal styles of Bagua zhang 八卦掌 (Eight Trigram Palm), Taiji quan 太極拳 (Great Ultimate Boxing), and Xingyi quan 形意拳 (Form Intent Boxing). It develops internal power and martial prowess, hardening the body by condensing *qi* in its external layers. One example is Iron Shirt Qigong, which involves hitting oneself with fists, paraphernalia (e.g., rice-filled socks), or external objects (e.g., trees) (see Chia 1986; Liang and Wu 1997, 237-77). Martial Qigong is frequently used as a supplement to formal martial arts training.

Medical Qigong is associated with TCM and sometimes prescribed as part of a treatment. It may be preventative or curative, maintaining health or working as a remedy. It enhances health, understood as the smooth flow of *qi* throughout the organ-meridian system, and eliminates disease, seen as excess, stagnation, or obstruction. There are innumerable preventative medical Qigong methods; they form the majority of exercises currently in circulation and advocated by practitioners (see Cohen 1997). With its key emphasis on health, vitality, and longevity, medical Qigong is a secular or at least transreligious practice, so that people of any religious or cultural background can benefit from it. Representative examples of curative medical Qigong include exercises aimed at specific medical conditions, such as spleen-*qi* deficiency, eye problems, and so forth (see Liang and Wu 1997, 23-75; J. A. Johnson 2000).

There are also martial and medical forms of Qigong that involve "issuing" or "emitting *qi*" (*faqi* 發氣). Martial practitioners use their in-

ner power to defeat an opponent, often through dramatic demonstrations wherein the person in question is thrown across a room or open
space. Medical adepts often practice external *qi*-healing, most commonly using intention and the Labor Palace (Laogong 勞宮; PC-8)
point in the center of the palm to send *qi* into another person (Cohen
1997, 242-64). This may be considered a form of therapeutic touch.
There are important precautions that must be taken when engaging
in external *qi*-healing to avoid transmitting toxins into the patient or
absorbing the patient's diseased *qi*.

The other two categories of Qigong, Buddhist and Daoist, are slightly
more problematic. Should one merely accept practitioners' self-
identification of the practices, or should one adopt a more skeptical
set of evaluative criteria? Should one define such forms of Qigong as
limited to those that originate in the respective traditions and are
practiced and advocated by adherents, or should one also include
those that merely claim affinities with certain religious worldviews?

Today few Qigong systems originate in Buddhist or Daoist contexts.
Some forms have mythological associations, Daoists and Buddhists
practice certain exercises, and Qigong groups are on occasion affili-
ated with religious communities, but in general religious links are
highly dubious. That is, few practitioners of Huashan Qigong (L.
Johnson 2001; 2002) or Wudang Qigong (Liu 1999) have trained at
these Daoist mountain monasteries or studied with their affiliates.
They have no lineage standing in a Daoist school and no formal training in these systems. In addition, the religious goals and ideals of
Daoism play little or no role in the practice, the main concern of Daoists often being on ritual and devotion rather than the physical component of the teachings. Thus, Min Zhiting 閔智亭 (1924-2004), former Chairman of the Chinese Daoist Association, in his manual on
Daoist monastic life makes no mention of Qigong (Min 1990). Similarly, in the recent *Taoism* (2002), published by the Chinese Daoist
Association, there are only two photographs of physical practice. This
English-language publication, written by Daoists, depicts Daoism as
a monastic, ritualistic, and meditative tradition.

Nevertheless, some Qigong systems are associated with Buddhist or
Daoist lineages, such as the Buddhist Shaolin Temple in Henan and
Mount Emei in Sichuan, as well as the Daoist Mount Hua in Shaanxi
and Mount Wudang in Hubei. From what we know today, most of
these exercises emerged in a secular, lay context and were later le-
gitimized through association with a well-known saint or famous sacred site. Buddhists thus have "Bodhidharma's Muscle Changing and

Marrow Cleansing Exercises" (see Yang 1989b; Cohen 1997, 194-99), linked with the first Chinese patriarch of Chan Buddhism, with Shaolin Temple, and with some *mūdras* (sacred gestures), but otherwise not particularly religious or Buddhist in nature.

There is, however, also Buddhist Qigong in the narrower sense. It utilizes Tantric views of the body together with *mūdras* and *mantras* (sacred sounds) and locates the practitioner within a context of *samsāra* and the search for liberation. It bears the influence of Indian Yogic and Tibetan Buddhist views and practices, as well as the belief in the sacred and magical power of Sanskrit seed syllables.[2] It can be described as a popular modification of more esoteric Buddhist practices, but its history is still unclear.[3]

Daoist Qigong is complex. There are many parallels between earlier longevity practices and modern Qigong forms. Breathing, healing exercises, and *qi*-absorption have played an important role in Daoist cultivation since the Highest Clarity movement of the fourth century. The main difference to modern forms is that traditional Daoist training used physical exercises mainly as a preparatory measure and in addition required dietary transformation, the taking of herbal and mineral drugs, prolonged periods of meditation, as well as a profound sense of devotion to the gods, skilled ritual performance, and a goal of complete transcendence.

Daoist Qigong as a form of practice that expresses specifically Daoist views and goals appears in certain systems, such as Healing Tao, that represent a simplification and popularization of inner alchemy (*neidan* 內丹) with its focus on the Three Treasures of vital essence (*jing* 精), *qi*, and spirit (*shen* 神); the three elixir fields (*dantian* 丹田); as well as activating the Daoist subtle body (see Liang and Wu 1997, 77-126; Chia 1993; Yang 2003). However, like the so-called Buddhist practices, it is unclear how many practitioners of such forms embrace a Daoist worldview or focus on Daoist goals, and often there is little evidence of the goal of rarification and self-divinization traditionally part of Daoist alchemical systems.

Moreover, it is not entirely clear what the referents for "immortality" are within Qigong communities. In many cases it seems that immortality becomes a code word for enlightenment, spiritual abilities,

---

[2] See Liang and Wu 1997, 127-73; also L. Johnson 1998; Newton 2001.

[3] Perhaps the most well-known form of contemporary Buddhist Qigong is Falun gong (Dharma Wheel Exercises). For emic presentations of this system, see www.falundafa.org; www.faluninfo.net.

and/or higher levels of consciousness. The same may be said concern-ing the concept of Dao. More often than not, contemporary Qigong practitioners place tradition-specific systems under the broader ru-bric of spiritual Qigong, creating their own mix of ideas and concepts in the process.

In addition to these four types, there are many modern forms that fall between the categories and show different characteristics. Some such Qigong systems, rooted in earlier longevity practices with compara-tively old pedigrees, include the Five Animal Frolics (*wuqin xi* 五禽戲), Six Healing Sounds (*liuzi jue* 六字訣), and Eight Brocades (*baduan jin* 八段錦). However, in the context of Qigong discourse, such historical details are often manipulated, intentionally or not, to create legiti-macy and authority, and thus power and increased economic prosper-ity. For example, in his book *The Way of Qigong*, Ken Cohen explains,

> *Baduan jin* means literally "Eight Pieces of Silk Brocade."
> These eight exercises are elegant, graceful, and essential
> methods of *qi*-cultivation. They were first described in an
> eighth-century Daoist text, *Xiuzhen shishu* (Ten Treatises
> on Restoring the Original Vitality) in the Daoist Canon.
> Daoist tradition attributes the exercises to one of the Eight
> Immortals of Chinese folklore, Chong Li-quan [Zhongli
> Quan]. (Cohen 1997, 186)

The form he refers to has two variants. The standing Eight Brocades, which are highly popular today, are nowhere to be found in tradi-tional literature, either Daoist or Buddhist (see Fig. 1). They may well be very recent. The seated Eight Brocades is a set of exorcistic and cleansing practices that involves stretches, devotional activation of body gods, and meditations that serve to prepare practitioners for inner alchemy practice. It is known today but not frequently done (see Olson 1997). The sequence indeed appears first in the *Xiuzhen shishu* 修真十書 (DZ 263, 19.4a-5b) and is linked with Zhongli Quan 鐘離權, but does not go back to the 700s. Rather, the text is an anonymous anthology compiled around 1300. This is just one example of many where modern practitioners latch on to bits and pieces of historical information and then replace accuracy with wishful thinking.

Beyond the four major types of Qigong, other classifications include distinctions between moving or active Qigong (*donggong* 動功) and tranquil or passive Qigong (*jinggong* 靜功), exercises that involve ex-ternal movements of the body versus methods that involve keeping the body still (Cohen 1997, 4; Reid 1998, 55-56). Active Qigong resembles exercise as conventionally understood, while tranquil Qigong is meditation.

A yet different way of categorizing is according to postures: walking/moving, standing, sitting, and lying down. Most modern forms fall into the walking and standing groups, while seated and lying down exercises are often described as Daoyin 導引 or traditional healing exercises and stillness practices are called meditation or "quiet sitting" (*jingzuo* 靜坐). However, as the Qigong movement unfolds, these practices find increasing integration into the larger spectrum. Their inclusion may well be an effective marketing strategy to increase appeal to wider segments of the population (see Palmer 2005; 2006).[4]

Finally, one may also categorize Qigong according to goals and levels of practice. Goals may include healing and preservation of health, stress relief and relaxation, longevity and youthfulness, strength building and martial prowess, spiritual cultivation and cosmological attunement, energetic awareness and mystical communion, and even immortality.

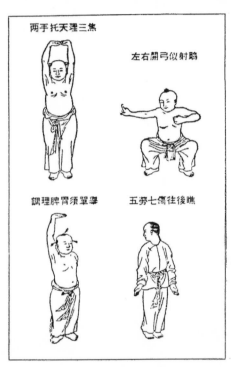

两手托天理三焦

左右開弓似射鵰

調理脾胃須單舉

五勞七傷往後瞧

Fig. 1: Standing Eight Brocades

---

[4] Another aspect of the market-oriented nature of Qigong and other American spiritual practices is the increased emergence of proprietorship, the culmination of commodification. For example, Dahn Yoga/Holistic Tao, a Korean syncretic spiritual system, like Bikram Yoga™, has trademarked its practices, which include Dahnhak® and Brain Respiration®™. Like the relationship of the Pepsi™ corporation to the Coca Cola™ corporation, this may represent an attempt to profit from the Healing Tao (Mantak Chia's system) brand name. Holistic Tao currently has over 360 centers in Korea, the United States, Canada, United Kingdom, Brazil, and Japan. See www.holistictao.com; www.dahnyoga.com.

From an anthropological and cultural studies perspective, these goals are more complex than they first appear and it is not entirely clear how various Qigong practitioners and communities understand concepts of health, disease, spirituality, and so forth (see Kleinman 1980; Unschuld 1985). Clearly the most influential presentations and the majority of Qigong practitioners focus on health and healing, but some see them as preliminary to more spiritual aspirations. These, however, are context-specific and the result of a wide variety of cultural influences that are all the more complex in contemporary American society characterized by globalization, multiculturalism, and religious pluralism.

Orientalist Legacies

Orientalism was brought to prominence as a critical category by Edward Said (1979). Although conventionally associated with the Western study of the Middle East, it may refer to any Western or European representation of Asian culture, in which artificial and wishful constructions come to hold primacy or interpretative authority. That is to say, in an Orientalist mode, the primary frame of reference is a radical dualism or bifurcation between the West and the East, the Occident and the Orient. As a pejorative or critical category, Orientalism may refer to Western discourse strategies that rely on a domination paradigm, in which Western representations are given priority over indigenous cultural realities, i.e., ethnic or national groups as well as religious and cultural traditions.[5]

Orientalism is first and foremost characterized by Western fantasies and is intimately bound to Western colonialism, whether political, military, or intellectual. Early Orientalist accounts of Asian cultures included seeing Asians as irrational, undeveloped, dangerous, exotic, sexualized, and so forth. Although these views are obviously outdated and inaccurate, various Orientalist legacies continue to frame discussions, appropriations, and transformations of Asian beliefs and prac-

---

[5] The corresponding phenomenon of "Occidentalism" (e.g., how Americans are represented in Chinese or Saudi Arabian culture) has yet to be adequately considered. The tendency toward vilification and demonization is a global phenomenon. As a counter-point to Iwamura's research on the Oriental monk (2000), an entire paper could be written on "the Occidental villain" in the context of various Asian or Middle Eastern cultures.

tices as well as relationships and interactions with people of Asian descent.

While earlier presentations of Asians most frequently depicted them as villains, one of the most prominent contemporary Orientalist constructs is that of the Oriental Monk (see Iwamura 2000; Siegler 2003). He is perceived by Westerners as an embodiment of spirituality and the hope for an alternative future, in which materialism is abandoned and spirituality retrieved. The Oriental Monk represents the ancient wisdom of the East and transmits it to a new cultural context, found in an idealized vision of "America" as a storehouse and safe haven for allegedly dying Eastern spiritual traditions. Some prominent examples include Kwai Chang Caine, Deepak Chopra, the Dalai Lama, Thich Nhat Hanh, Mr. Migayi, and D. T. Suzuki (see Iwamura 2000). In terms of Chinese cultural traditions in America, one finds the Oriental Monk as "Daoist Master," "Qigong Master," or "Taiji Master," sometimes even self-described as "Grand Master" (J. A. Johnson 2000, 1029).

Qigong practitioners and self-identified Daoists in America tend to rely on this enduring Orientalist legacy to establish and increase their cultural capital. Especially in terms of Daoism, they appropriate popular (and often faulty) representations and use psychological sensitivity to create spiritualist businesses. Even a cursory perusal of popular American publications, an internet search of "Taoism" and "Daoism," or conversations with leading representatives reveal that the Daoism of the popular Western imagination has very little in common with the historical contours of the Chinese Daoist tradition (see Kirkland 1997; Siegler 2003).

For example, almost any issue of *The Empty Vessel*, a popular quarterly journal on "contemporary American Taoism," shows Daoism in the United States to be closer to a form of New Age spirituality or perennial philosophy than the complex religious tradition of China.[6] American Daoism centers on the ideas of the *Daode jing*, translated

---

[6] "Perennial philosophy" is a term originally coined by Gottfried Wilhelm von Leibniz and conceptually developed by Aldous Huxley (1946). It claims that all the major mystical systems of the world share the same "perennial" worldview: that the phenomenal world is partially real, being a secondary manifestation of an underlying Ground; that human beings can know the Ground by direct intuition; that they are divided into a conscious ego and an eternal true self; and that it is the chief end of human existence to discover and become one with the true self as Ground. See Happold 1970, 20.

in popularized versions that have increasingly less to do with the original and are interpreted to fit the modern American mind (see LaFargue and Pas 1998). Daoism is packaged in a form that conforms to dominant cultural assumptions and desires and is thus more easily appropriated and marketed. As Solala Towler says:

> [Daoism] goes back thousands of years, to a time before or-ganized religion, before ideologies overcame philosophy. It goes back to a time when humankind was not disconnected from the natural world, when humans learned from both the animal and the vegetable kingdom. . . . True Taoism is not an ideology or a New Age movement, it is a living phi-losophy. It is a way of thinking, a way of looking at life, a way of being; being *with* change rather than against it. It is a way of utilizing the natural energy of our bodies and minds in a healthy and graceful way. (Towler 1996, vii; 1998; also Blofeld 1973, 13)

Daoism in the American mind has therefore become a philosophy that predates organized religion, an ancient, universal wellspring for each and every Chinese health and spiritual tradition. It is responsible for numerous practices, such as TCM, Fengshui, *Yijing* divination, Taiji quan, and Qigong that are not Daoist in origin or essence, but appro-priated for a greater mystique and enhanced marketing potential. Daoism also ceases to be "a foreign path" and Americans do not need to become "Pseudo-Asians" (Towler 1996, viii)—yet every teacher mentioned in Towler's subsequent presentation is a Chinese immi-grant or Chinese American. That is, on one level Daoism is a univer-sal wisdom tradition that transcends culture, while on another only people of Chinese descent represent "true Daoism": once again, as per the Orientalist discourse, Chineseness is a requirement for authentic-ity.

Orientalism pervades the way Daoism is seen in the Qigong commu-nity. Within the American Qigong movement there are a variety of misconceptions, with some of the most prominent and influential be-ing the following:

- There is an original, pure Daoism, often called "philosophical Dao-ism."

- The hoary sage of antiquity named Laozi founded it.

- The *Daode jing* is the "Daoist bible."

- Daoism is non-theistic and means going with the flow.

- Daoist identity is something that one wears on the outside.

- All Daoists are nature-lovers.

- Chineseness is equivalent to authenticity.

In addition, there is a conflation of Fengshui, Qigong, Taiji quan, and TCM with Daoism. Daoism—thoroughly colonized and domesticated—is thereby easily adapted to Western and New Age sensibilities and, of course, becomes highly marketable to American consumers.[7]

Early American Masters

The Communist take-over of China in 1949 and the Cultural Revolution (1966-1976) caused the migration and forced exile of Chinese cultural elites, many of whom came to the United States, aided by the liberalization of American immigration laws in 1965. Many of them were trained in martial arts, Taiji quan, or Daoism and began to teach their practices in *dōjōs* and medical establishments, contributing to the budding Qigong movement.

DA LIU (1904-2000) began his study of Taiji quan under Sun Lutang 孫祿堂 (1861-1932),[8] the founder of the Sun style. Later he traveled to China's southwest provinces, where he trained with a number of teachers and became a practitioner of the Yang style. In 1955 he came to America and began teaching Taiji quan classes in New York City. During the late 1950s and early 1960s, he made several television appearances and his story, together with information about Taiji quan, appeared in many newspapers and magazines.

He also became president of the T'ai Chi Society of New York (www.chutaichi.com) and wrote a number of books on Taiji quan and other longevity practices (1972; 1974; 1978; 1979). The books present an integrated training program for health and long life with Taiji quan identified as primary. They include some of the earliest English-language accounts of classic Qigong forms, such as the Eight Brocades and the Five Animal Frolics. They also exerted some influence

---

[7] For more details on the role and history of Daoism in America, see Komjathy 2003a; 2003b; 2004; Siegler 2003. For reliable introductions to Daoism see Kohn 2001; Miller 2003; Kirkland 2004. For guidance on accurate electronic resources see www.daoistcenter.org.

[8] Whenever known, Chinese characters are included in the first appearance of a given teacher's name.

on the later publications of Stuart Olson (1997; 2002a) and Yang Jwing-ming (1989a; 1989b), two central figures in American Qigong.

T. T. LIANG (Tung-tsai Liang; 1900-2002), a former customs official, moved to the United States in 1963. A senior disciple of Zheng Man-qing 鄭曼青 (Cheng Man-ch'ing; 1901-1975), a leader of the Yang school of Taiji quan, he became an independent teacher, living first in Boston and later in Minnesota and teaching mainly in parks rather than in an organized studio. He popularized Taiji quan (Liang 1977) and taught some prominent teachers, including Stuart Olson (www.valleytaichi.com; Olson 2002b) and Paul Gallagher (www.totaltaichi.com).

LILY SIOU (a.k.a. Chang Yi Hsiang; b. 1945?), unlike Da Liu and T. T. Liang who were first and foremost Taiji quan instructors, specifically taught Qigong and published the first English book on the subject (1973). Allegedly a direct successor of the Celestial Master, a major leader of traditional, ritual Daoism, she founded the School of the Six Chinese Arts in Honolulu, Hawaii in 1970. The school was formally registered in 1972, received state accreditation as a Chinese medical school in 1976, was nationally accredited in 1991, and is now called the World Medicine Institute (acupuncture-hi.com).

As she says in the preface of her book, which was popular enough to go through four reprints: "Through it [this book], I hope to show the way to better health and well-being through the natural movements of Ch'i Kung," which is "an ancient but profound body and mind discipline, embodying much of Chinese philosophy." The work is quite eclectic, covering Chinese cosmology, Chinese medical theories and herbology, as well as some aspects of Daoism and the martial arts.

From Siou's perspective, Qigong predates Daoism and is best defined as "an ancient art of breath control based on the early Tao philosophy but predating the Taoists. Ch'i Kung is practiced in its pure form by the Taoists and in its secondary forms of T'ai Ch'i Ch'uan and Kung Fu Boxing by martial arts" (1973, 33). She goes on to discuss various aspects of Qigong practice, including principles, general sensations, personal experiences, and organ function. The third section of the book contains illustrated instruction on two exercise systems identified as the seated and standing Eight Brocades. The book concludes with archival photographs of the School of the Six Chinese Arts, including its members and activities.

The "Six Chinese/Taoist arts" in the name of Siou's school are ritual, music, archery, charioteering, writing, and mathematics—the classical arts of the Confucian gentleman in ancient China (acupuncture-hi.com/6arts.shtml; Siou 1973, 31).[9] According to Siou, Zhang Enpu 張恩溥, the 63rd Celestial Master, transmitted his lineage to her at Mount Longhu 龍虎山 in 1969, and the "Heavenly Masters and Taoists of Lunghu shan are renowned throughout China for their expertise in the Six Taoist Arts of the Chou Dynasty" (acupuncture-hi.com/history.shtml).[10] At the present time, it is unclear how this construction of Daoism functions in the curriculum and community of her school, a major Chinese medical college in Hawaii. Like Yosan University (www.yosan.edu), which was founded by Ni Hua-ching and his sons in Los Angeles, it represents a conflation of TCM with Daoism, typical for the United States. One of her senior disciples, Roger Jahnke of the Health Action Clinic in Santa Barbara, moreover, is both a Chinese medical practitioner and a central figure in American Qigong.

B. P. CHAN (Bun Piac Chan; 1922-2002) arrived in New York City in 1974. He originally came as a visiting instructor to the William C. C. Chen School of T'ai Chi (www.williamccchen.com), where he first taught Bagua zhang and later Xingyi quan and Chen-style Taiji quan.

---

[9] In Siou's construction, these "six arts" are not understood literally but metaphorically. For example, "charioteering" is said to symbolize the discipline and cultivation of the mind, body, and spirit, and to relate to the ability to harness, control, and direct *qi* (acupuncture-hi.com/charioteering.shtml).

[10] This is unlikely for a wide variety of reasons. First, no female priest has ever held the position of Celestial Master (it is a patriarchal and patrilineal position). Second, Siou's timeline contradicts historical facts; Zhang Enpu died before Siou claims the transmission occurred. Finally, the Celestial Masters lineage, in fact, passed from Zhang Enpu to Zhang Yuanxian 張源先(64th Celestial Master) and then to Zhang Jiyu 張繼禹 (65th), the current lineage holder. The latter two have published histories of the Celestial Masters movement (Ding 2000, 775).

Other equally questionable characters on the American Daoist scene are Kwan Sai-hung and Liu Ming. Kwan Sai-hung, the central figure in the "Wandering Taoist" trilogy (see Deng 1993), which is possibly the first American Daoist hagiography, claims to be a Chinese immigrant and to have received extensive training at Huashan. However, preliminary research suggests that he was actually born in New York City and that *Chronicles of Tao* was largely based on various other sources, including Morrison's *Hua Shan* (1974; Anderson 1989). Likewise, Liu Ming, the founder of Orthodox Daoism in America, most often appears in public in full Daoist robes and a top-knot, while making frequent claims about "Daoist orthodoxy." And yet, there is no evidence that he was ordained, and, in fact, the recent disbandment of his ODA Seattle parish centered on his inability to produce the ordination certificate or the texts upon which his authority as a self-identified Daoist priest rest.

Within a year, he decided to remain in the United States and continued to teach in William Chen's community for the next twenty-seven years (see Cohen 2002a). He is significant as one of the first to teach Taiji chi 太極尺 (Taiji Ruler), a Qigong form that utilizes an hourglass shaped wooden stick.[11] He learned this form from Zhao Zhongdao 趙中道 (1844-1962), the founder of the Supple Art of Taiji Health Society in Beijing and the first to teach Taiji Ruler publicly (Cohen 2002b). Chan is also important as one of the main teachers of Ken Cohen, an important figure in American Qigong today.

MANTAK CHIA (Xie Mingde 謝明德; b. 1944) has exerted perhaps the greatest influence through his enduring institution of Healing Tao/Dao. Born in Thailand to Chinese parents, he practiced Buddhist meditation from the age of six and soon after met his first Taiji quan teacher, a certain Master Lu. Later, when he was a student in Hong Kong, a classmate named Cheng Sue-sue introduced him to his first Daoist teacher, Yi Eng 一雲 (One Cloud). At this point, he began serious Daoist training and learned various cultivation methods, such as the Microcosmic Orbit, Fusion of the Five Elements, and inner alchemy. "It was Yi Eng who authorized Master Chia to teach and heal" (Chia 1993, xiii).

After training with other teachers, including Mui Yimwattana, Cheng Yao-lun, and Pan Yu, Chia combined his knowledge of Daoism and the other disciplines to formulate the Healing Tao system. In 1974 he established the Natural Healing Center in Thailand, and five years later moved to New York City. Since then, Healing Tao centers have opened in many other locations throughout North America, Europe, and Asia. It is an international organization and a global Qigong practice. In addition, Mantak Chia has published numerous books (e.g., 1983; 1985; 1986; 1993) (www.healingtaousa.com). Chia's system is

---

[11] An earlier Qigong system called "T'ai Chi Chih" and created by Justin Stone (1996) has certain characteristics that resemble Taiji Ruler, but there are major deviations and the distinctive wooden ruler is not mentioned. Stone created this series of twenty exercises in 1974, based on "several little-known movements [learned] from an old Chinese man" (1996, 12). He explains that the "T'ai Chi Chih" of the title means "knowledge of the supreme ultimate." This may be a confusion of *chih* 知 ("knowledge") for *ch'ih* 尺 ("ruler"). Stone's system has a large following in the United States; by 1996, he had accredited about 1,100 instructors (1996, 13; Cohen 2002b).

sometimes also called "Tao Yoga," "Taoist Yoga," or "Taoist Esoteric Yoga" (Chia 1983).[12]

At some point, Chia moved back to Thailand, where he currently lives and teaches at the Tao Garden Health Resort (www.tao-garden.com) and runs a new variation of the Healing Tao System called Universal Tao (www.universal-tao.com). He has trained a large number of senior instructors (www.taoinstructors.org), and Healing Tao USA has continued to thrive and expand under the leadership of Michael Winn (b. 1951), also at one time president of the National Qigong Association. Healing Tao USA is now a private educational trust in the process of filing for non-profit status. It operates Healing Tao University at the Jeronimo Center (New York), a set of summer workshops and seminars, as well as the website and fulfillment center.

The practice system of Healing Tao contains a structured set of inner alchemy practices, which may represent a distinctively American form, and involves a wide range of certifications (www.healingtaousa.com; www.healingdao.com). It combines practices according to a version developed by Michael Winn and includes seven alchemy formulas of immortality as transmitted from Yi Eng to Mantak Chia. After practicing the foundational practice of the Inner Smile, one progresses through the following stages: (1) Open the Orbit, Five Phases of Spirit and Eight Extraordinary Vessels; (2) Lesser Enlightenment of Water and Fire; (3) Greater Enlightenment of Water and Fire; (4) Greatest Enlightenment of Water and Fire; (5) Sealing the Senses; (6) Congress of Heaven and Earth; and (7) Union of Man and Dao.[13]

T. K. SHIH (Shih Tzu-kuo 施祖果; b. 1929), a doctor of Chinese medicine, immigrated to New York City in the late 1970s. In the early 1980s, he founded the Chinese Healing Arts Center (www.qihealer.com) and the Wu Tang Ch'üan Association in Kingston, which identifies some of its practices as originating at the Daoist sacred site of Mount

---

[12] This is, of course, historically inaccurate. Yoga is a Sanskrit term meaning "to yoke" and by extension "to unite;" it refers to a diverse set of Indian spiritual systems with divergent goals. While Daoist inner alchemy has certain similarities with Kundalini and Tantric Yoga (which both Chia and Winn have practiced), and while Chinese long life practices find parallels in Hatha Yoga, there is no such thing as "Daoist Yoga." How these practices came to be so identified remains unknown, but one of the earliest occurrences is Lu K'uan-yü's *Taoist Yoga* (1970), the translation of a Qing-dynasty manual of inner alchemy.

[13] For more information on Healing Tao see Belamide 2000; Komjathy 2003a; 2003b; 2004; Siegler 2003.

Wudang. T. K. Shih has published two books on Qigong (1989; 1994), the former of which is the earliest English-language publication on the Swimming Dragon, an exercise for opening the spine and moistening the connective tissue. It is also praised as "the unique Chinese way to fitness, beautiful skin, weight loss, and high energy." Beyond its medical benefits, Qigong here for the first time is lauded as having the power to facilitate weight loss and increase beauty.

Like Michael Winn, T. K. Shih frequently takes out full-page advertisements in the opening pages of *The Empty Vessel*. In a recent issue (Spring 2005), Shih offers workshops and seminars on seasonal cooking, Swimming Dragon practice, as well as Qi Healer and Qigong Therapist training at various levels. In terms of contemporary developments, this advertisement is representative of a larger trend in contemporary American Qigong: professionalization. Under this logic, to be an authentic Qigong teacher requires certification and accreditation, which is, of course, a way of maintaining and strengthening personal authority as well as an excellent marketing strategy.

YANG JWING-MING 楊俊敏 (b. 1946) came to the United States from Taiwan in 1974 to pursue an engineering degree at Purdue University. Having trained in the martial arts from the age of fifteen, and despite his successful conclusion of the Ph. D., he decided to become a martial arts teacher. In 1982, he established Yang's Martial Arts Association (YMAA) in Boston, where he teaches everything from Shaolin Long Fist and White Crane Gongfu to Yang-style Taiji quan, Xingyi quan, and Bagua zhang (www.ymaa.com).

He has also become a prolific author of over fifty videos and thirty books, including nine on Qigong (1985; 1988; 1989a; 1989b; 2003). While there is a great deal of repetition throughout these publications, he generally makes a distinction among different types of Qigong, including martial, medical, Daoist, and Buddhist. In addition to covering Qigong theory, Yang's books provide illustrated instruction on specific practices, including the standing Eight Brocades and tendon-changing and marrow-washing exercises. Like the earlier publications of Da Liu, Stephan Chang (1978), and others, Yang Jwing-ming also provides illustrations of the organ-meridian networks often utilized in both medical and Daoist forms of Qigong (Yang 1989a, 200-41). Here one may identify an "alternative" understanding of the body and embodiment, at least partially based on subtle energetic networks.

CHEN HUI-XIAN (b. 1933) represents the final stage of the early transmission of Qigong to the United States. An interpreter for the Chinese Ministry of Foreign Trade and later a university English teacher,

Chen developed lymphatic cancer in 1982, when she was forty-nine years old. Doctors gave her a twenty-five percent chance of recovery. While waiting for chemotherapy and radiation treatment in a Beijing clinic, a fellow patient told her about a Qigong form that had helped cure him of cancer. This was Soaring Crane Qigong (Hexiang zhuang 鶴翔狀), developed and taught by Zhao Jinxiang 趙金香 (b. 1934) in Beijing parks. After three months of intensive daily practice under the direction of Zhao, Chen regained her health (Towler 1996, 4-7). Following her recovery, she decided that her life mission was to spread Soaring Crane Qigong throughout the world.

Around 1985, Chen moved to Portland and began teaching Qigong at the Oregon College of Oriental Medicine (www.ocom.edu). She also initiated a teacher-certification program, which has gained increasing standing in contemporary American Qigong. In addition to writing a number of self-published manuals on Soaring Crane (Chen and Alswel 1995; Chen 1996), Chen founded the Wu Dao Jing She International Society of Qigong in 1996 with Charles Wu, through which she has trained and certified many prominent American Qigong teachers, including Solala Towler (www.wudaojingshe.com). Aside from being the main representative of Soaring Crane Qigong in America, Chen Hui-xian is also representative of another major trend in the Qigong movement, namely the effort at self-healing, especially of serious medical conditions. In this she is like other major figures who healed themselves through Qigong: Jiang Weiqiao of tuberculosis, Liu Guizhen of a stomach ulcer, Guo Lin of cancer, T. K. Shih of tuberculosis, and Solala Towler of chronic fatigue syndrome (see Miura 1989; Palmer 2005; 2006). That is, many of the originators of Qigong systems and major proponents of certain Qigong exercises turned personal journeys toward health into life-missions.

The relationship among disease, healing, and health comes into sharper focus from such personal testimonials. One prominent Qigong ideal is enduring health, a life free from disease. One might assume that followers interpret disease as failure or deficiency. While this is the case *after* one has practiced Qigong, it is not true *before* one has begun such training. Instead, disease becomes a sign that one's life is out of balance; disease is a call to change. In short, for many, illness initiates a conversion process that results in becoming practitioners, teachers, and advocates.

Key Characteristics

From these brief biographical sketches certain characteristics of the early phase of Qigong in America become clear. The American Qigong movement emerged through the lives and teachings of Chinese immigrants. Most began teaching in New York City in the 1970s and 1980s. Tentatively speaking, one may identify the demographics of the early American Qigong movement as follows: an individual Chinese immigrant teacher surrounded by mainly white middle-class students, many of whom became second-generation teachers. In this way, Qigong in America parallels similar American appropriations of "Eastern spiritual technologies" (e.g., Buddhist meditation, Tibetan Tantra, Yoga, etc.) as well as developments in the New Age movement more generally.

As a secular Chinese health and longevity practice, Qigong was also easily assimilated into the American health and fitness movement, so much so that T. K. Shih speaks of the Swimming Dragon as a method for weight loss and beauty enhancement. Similarly, because of its emphasis on health and healing, Qigong also joined the emerging American interest in "alternative medicine." As we have seen, many of the early teachers and proponents of Qigong began practicing Qigong to heal themselves and in response to the failure of allopathic medicine. One might, in turn, read Qigong practice as an implicit critique of modernization and industrialization, even though many Qigong teachers speak of the practice in modern medical and scientific terms.

In addition, the early American Qigong movement revolved around a relatively small repertoire of exercises: Eight Brocades, Five Animal Frolics, Soaring Crane, Swimming Dragon, and Taiji Ruler. Often teachers only taught one of these forms. Nonetheless, they all had a certain amount of cultural capital because they originated in China and since students had very little previous knowledge. Some teachers had older pedigrees, while others emerged during the Qigong boom that swept through China in the 1980s. The early history of Qigong in America, moreover, also corresponds to the early history of Westernized "Daoism," Taiji quan, and TCM. In these years, there were few or no practice centers specifically dedicated to Qigong. Instead, it was taught at martial *dōjōs*, Taiji quan academies, and TCM colleges. It was and is also one of the primary ways that self-identified American Daoists make a living in the context of American capitalism.

The present account of the early history of Qigong in America has certain omissions that should be recognized. First, there is a heavy emphasis on the lives of specific teachers. At the present time, it is unclear how the early communities were organized, how many people participated, and what their motivations were. One also could reasonably argue that the popularity of Qigong derived as much from the early publications as the early practitioners. Similarly, while I have mentioned certain historical events that played some role in the early transmission of Qigong in America, there are, of course, many other factors involved, including the loosening of restrictions on Chinese immigration following the Immigration Act of 1965 and a growing interest in complementary medicine and alternative spirituality.

In terms of bringing Chinese medicine and other Chinese health practices to American attention, one key event was President Richard Nixon's visit to China in 1971, during which *New York Times* columnist James Reston recovered from an appendectomy with the help of acupuncture anesthesia. The present account also leaves out the personal histories of those who became the second-generation of American Qigong teachers. While some of these individuals studied with the teachers mentioned above, others, such as B. K. Frantzis (www.energyarts.com), Mark Johnson (www.chi-kung.com), and Daniel Reid (Taiwan), went to China or Taiwan in search of teachers and to deepen their understanding and practice. That is, in addition to early Chinese immigrant teachers, the early history of Qigong in America is also the story of pilgrimages to the East. For example, Mark Johnson when living and studying in Taiwan met Ni Hua-ching, one of the most influential early self-identified Daoist teachers in America, and arranged for him to teach at the Taoist Sanctuary (then in Los Angeles) (Siegler 2003; Komjathy 2004).

Contemporary American Qigong

Since the late 1980s, Qigong in America has become increasingly popular. With each passing year, more books are published, more teachers emerge, more centers are being established, and more people have become practitioners.[14] Today, Qigong is so much a part of popu-

---

[14] The recent explosion of Qigong teachers proves challenging for older and more established teachers. As expressed by Yang Jwing-ming, "So many students in America are going around calling themselves Master. Many of them don't even practice themselves, how can they call themselves Master?

lar American culture that one can find teachers and centers in most urban areas. A recent Internet search on a major search-engine under "Chi Kung" resulted in over 440,000 hits, while the same search under "Qigong" resulted in over 650,000 hits. A similar search of books in print yields between 500 and 8,000 titles under "Chi Kung" and about 200 titles under "Qigong," including several specifically for women (Ferraro 2000; Y. L. Johnson 2001). Granted, these are less than scientific findings, but they, like similar searches through local telephone directories (e.g., Douglas 2002, 285-312), reveal just how widespread and how well-established Qigong practice is in the U.S.

A systematic account of American Qigong, composed of a diverse group of teachers, students, practices, and communities, would require a book-length study. Unlike the previous section on the early history of Qigong in America, which focused on early immigrant Chinese teachers, this section discusses the contemporary situation, the most prominent and influential organizations as well as some of its general characteristics.

First of all, the increasing popularity of Qigong in America has led to major shifts in the composition and focus of the movement. While Chinese immigrant teachers, especially those who have come to the United States more recently, continue to play a role, the majority of teachers and students are now Euro-Americans. In addition, market factors of supply and demand have created certain unforeseen opportunities: it is now possible to make a living as a Qigong instructor. This, in turn, has resulted in a new stratification.

Qigong teachers today operate on various societal levels: national, regional, and local. There is an emphasis on visibility, growth, and group size as indicative of success. Quantity of publications, numbers of students, and public prominence often supersede quality of instruction and depth of understanding. Where in traditional settings personal affinity with a teacher, the teacher's level of understanding, and personal experience of the system were paramount, now many within the Qigong movement harbor ambitions for greater recognition, influence, and economic prosperity. They find themselves contending and competing for status and resources both within Qigong as well as in the general area of complementary health care and alternative spirituality. As national Qigong organizations emerge and grow, to be known and wealthy is to be successful.

This kind of thing discourages traditional Chinese Masters to teach American students" (Towler 1996, 25).

Among the various levels of presence, without dismissing the cumulative effect and the contribution to individual lives made by local practitioners, national teachers and organizations are clearly the most visible and influential. They include:

- Effie Chow of the East West Academy of the Healing Arts (www.eastwestqi.com)
- Ken Cohen of the Qigong Research and Practice Center (www.qigonghealing.com)
- B. K. (Bruce Kumar) Frantzis of Energy Arts (www.energyarts. com)
- Roger Jahnke of the Institute of Integral Qigong and Tai Chi (www. feeltheqi.com)
- Jerry Alan Johnson of the International Institute of Medical Qigong (www.qigong medicine.com)
- Mark Johnson of the Tai Chi for Health Institute (www.chi-kung.com)
- Solala Towler of the Abode of the Eternal Tao (www.abodetao.com)
- Michael Winn of Healing Tao USA (www.healingtaousa.com)
- Yang Jwing-ming of Yang's Martial Arts Association (www. ymaa.com)

Without going into biographical details and without disrespecting their personal experiences, they represent certain ideal types within the broader Qigong movement, which I would propose to call traditionalists, medicalists, spiritualists, and positivists.

Traditionalists (e.g., Ken Cohen) teach Qigong systems with older pedigrees, claim lineage connections with Chinese teachers, have knowledge of Chinese culture, and often wear Chinese clothing as a sign of their solidarity with things Chinese. They often identify themselves as Daoists. Medicalists (e.g., Jerry Alan Johnson, Roger Jahnke) teach preventative and restorative Qigong forms, often hold degrees in Chinese medicine, and frequently oversee and/or teach at TCM schools.

Spiritualists (e.g., Solala Towler, Michael Winn) identify Qigong as a form of spiritual (not religious) work, combining aspects from various religious traditions into a hybrid spirituality that has clear parallels with the characteristics of New Age spirituality and perennial philosophy outlined below, however much representatives resist such characterizations. Spiritualists frequently make claims about the connection between Qigong and "Daoism," with the latter stripped to a large extent of its historical and religious characteristics.

Positivists (e.g., Effie Chow, Roger Jahnke, Yang Jwing-ming), finally, interpret Qigong in terms of a modern Western scientific paradigm, often citing clinical and experimental studies that measure *qi* as electro-magnetism or that scientifically validate the health benefits and therapeutic success of Qigong.[15] Their validation goes beyond personal testimonials to recognition by Western biomedicine and science with roots in Cartesian dualism and mechanistic organicism. They understand Qigong as a secular or quasi-secular health practice, which transcends religious affiliations and can be supported by scientific research.

The dramatic growth of popular interest in Qigong throughout the 1990s has also resulted in the formation of national membership organizations. The most prominent umbrella organizations include:

- American Qigong Association (AQA; www.eastwestqi.com/aqa)

- National Qigong Association (NQA; www.nqa.org)

- Qigong Alliance (QA; www.qigong-alliance.org)

- Qigong Association of America (QAA; www.qi.org)

- World Qigong Federation (www.eastwestqi.com/wqf)

Of these, the National Qigong Association is the largest, most representative, and most influential. NQA was founded in 1995 (Jahnke 2005), and most prominent Qigong teachers in America have at one time or another served as presidents and chairmen.[16] NQA is a grassroots, nonprofit organization of Qigong practitioners working toward the following main goals:

---

[15] Qigong represents an "alternative" cultural practice that cannot be easily domesticated into modern biomedicine, although new research in biology and physics is developing a language that may make cross-cultural communication more possible. On scientific studies of Qigong see Cohen 1997; Jahnke 1999; 2002.

[16] The founders of NQA included James MacRitchie, Russell DesMarais, Berkeley Freeman, Jesse Dammann, Roger Jahnke, Damaris Jarboux, Mark Johnson, Richard Leirer, and Gunther Weil. The following individuals have been NQA president: James MacRitchie (1996), Russell DesMarais (1997), Michael Winn (1998; 1999), Solala Towler (2000; 2001), Jim Concotelli (2002), Malvin Finkelstein (2002; 2003), Shoshanna Katzman (2004), and Bonnitta Roy (2005). There also have been a variety of chairmen, some of whom include Francesco (Garri) Garripolli, Roger Jahnke, Michael DeMolina, and Gunther Weil.

1. To promote the principles and practices of Qigong.

2. To establish and integrate Qigong into all aspects of mainstream culture, healing, science, and education.

3. To encourage self-healing and spiritual self-development through daily Qigong practice.

4. To create a forum and network for sharing information about Qigong.

5. To unify classical and contemporary branches, schools and traditions of Qigong.

6. To assure the transference of the essence of Qigong between the East and West.

7. To integrate medical Qigong into the health care community.

8. To create, explore and establish unique forms of American Qigong.

9. To provide training for the public, students and practitioners of Qigong.

10. To foster peace and harmony throughout the world through Qigong principles and practices. (www.nqa.org)

NQA currently has about 700 members, organizes an annual conference, and provides online assistance for locating Qigong teachers and organizations. It has also sponsored an online Qigong journal entitled *The Journal of Qigong in America*, first issued in 2004 under the editorship of Michael Meyer.

Another major development on the national stage is the formation of the World T'ai Chi and Qigong Day (WTCQD). Bill Douglas, author of *The Complete Idiot's Guide to T'ai Chi and Qigong* (2002, orig. 1999), began this worldwide event in 1999. It begins each year at 10 a.m. local time on the Saturday of the week of United Nations World Health Day (April 29, 2006). In the United States, events are held in each of the fifty states. Local teachers and members of Qigong centers practice with an awareness of "the Day," and many teachers actively promote the event by opening their schools to the general public. There are also larger gatherings held in parks, during which practitioners introduce Taiji quan and Qigong to the larger public. Events range from small group sessions to massive public events, involving many teachers, practitioners, groups, and schools practicing in the same area. The motivation behind the event is to create a unique global health and healing celebration (Douglas 2002, 279-83; www.worldtaichiday.org).

The New Age Connection

What, then, accounts for the rising popularity of Qigong in America? One reason is obviously its greater visibility. Qigong has become increasingly accessible. In addition to many teachers and centers, there are numerous instructional resources, including books and articles as well as audio tapes, videos, and DVDs. Moreover, Qigong has been the subject of mainstream accounts, among them most importantly the 1993 PBS special *Healing and the Mind* by Bill Moyers, whose episode "The Mystery of Chi" documents the practice of Qigong in Chinese parks as well as external *qi* healing (N. Chen 2003, 28). Another Public Television documentary, *Qigong: Ancient Chinese Healing for the 21st Century*, was produced by Garri (Francesco) Garripoli and aired in 2001 (1999, 259-90; www.wujiproductions.com).

Another reason is that Qigong promises personal health and healing. Like Yoga, Taiji quan, TCM, and other Eastern arts, it fits into the larger contours of the American health and fitness movement and the search for alternative remedies (see Lau 2000; Roof 2001). As American health care sinks more deeply into crisis, fewer individuals and families can afford it. As patients find themselves more and more shackled by managed care, they grow increasingly skeptical of the motivations of physicians and the healthcare industry, whose research and products are largely funded by pharmaceutical companies (see Abramson 2004).

Qigong provides an alternative to the tendency of allopathic medicine to alienate individuals from their own personal experience, to view and treat the person as a machine with removable and replaceable parts, and to respond to disease along militaristic lines utilizing drugs with questionable results and serious side-effects. In contrast, the practice of Qigong emphasizes direct personal experience, focusing on both actual physicality and energetic layers of being. It provides people with a different kind of experience and practice, is much less invasive and more affordable, has positive effects, and results in personal benefits. Many practitioners find themselves more relaxed and having increased energy (Cohen 1997, 270-73). Joining a group for training and practice, many people also develop a feeling of belonging, which gives a greater sense of meaning in their lives. In contrast, few American Qigong teachers discuss possible dangers of Qigong practice, such as addiction and psychosis (see N. Chen 2003; also Cohen 1997, 273-78).

A third reason for the popularity of Qigong is that it is easily adaptable to the needs and desires of practitioners. It most frequently centers on health and fitness, complementary medicine, and alternative spirituality. Like the predominant American constructions of Daoism, Qigong matches the general characteristics of the New Age movement, which are as follows:

- Most New Age thought is essentially neo-Platonic. Adherents see all of existence as interconnected and all of the many levels of reality as forms of absolute Oneness.

- The Oneness of life can be discovered experientially in the depths of one's self. The essence of selfhood is divine.

- While most humans have forgotten this inner divinity, New Age adherents stress that it is possible to overcome these limitations and wrong ideas. For this, various spiritual technologies may be utilized.

- For New Agers, direct experience is what is authoritative, not the dictates of established tradition or the opinions of others. Daily decisions are made, not by obeying externally imposed commandments, but by following one's own intuition, inner guidance, and wisdom.

- Although New Agers are adverse to the authority of institutionalized or established religious traditions, they nonetheless feel free to draw upon those traditions as resources to create an eclectic and unique synthesis of various perspectives and practices.

- Most New Age adherents are perennialists. They believe that it is necessary to penetrate the external, superficial crust of religious dogmas and rituals—the differences that divide—in order to discover the universal core of hidden wisdom, the mystical essence that underlies all religions.

- New Age thought and practice is focused on transformation and healing (understood broadly), both for the individual and for the planet. By transforming and healing themselves, New Agers believe that they are helping to transform and heal the world around them.[17]

---

[17] For discussions of the New Age movement, see Barnard 2001, 311-13; also Lewis and Melton 1992; Hanegraaff 1998.

The similarities with popular American publications on Qigong, Daoism, and the like are obvious. Like the New Age movement, Qigong is easily incorporated into Protestant-influenced conceptions of non-religious spirituality. It is individualistic, simple and easy, anti-clerical and anti-ritualistic. There are no demands or requirements for membership, and one can benefit as much from personal daily practice as from workshops, seminars, and group sessions. In addition, the seemingly nebulous nature of Dao and *qi* allow them to become almost anything for anyone. In short, Qigong is easily marketable and easily consumable.

Conclusion

Qigong is the embodied practice of universal energies for the sake of healing and/or spirituality. "Embodiment" means a lived experience in which the body and physicality are given primacy of place. The fact that Western culture is in need of such a concept reveals just how systemic philosophical dualism has become.[18] In fact, there is no activity which does not involve the body, which is not "embodied," and the practice of Qigong should not be anything particular or special.

Still, embodiment is a useful metaphor to look at the American scene. It is what one's life represents, what is expressed through one's being and physical presence. Seen from this perspective, different people in the Qigong movement embody different things. Many prominent and influential teachers are individuals who began Qigong as a personal search for health. They became teachers through a sincere interest in helping others and embody a commitment to self-healing and altruism. Others began Qigong as a way to create and maintain identity. They became teachers in an attempt to gain power and authority and embody a commitment to self-aggrandizement and egoism. Yet others began Qigong as an opportunity to become recognized. They became teachers to profit from such recognition and embody a commitment to economic success and materialism. The intentions and motivations as well as goals and rhetorical strategies of American Qigong leaders are thus as varied as their life-stories and the exercises they advocate.

Their followers similarly practice Qigong for a variety of reasons: from maintaining and restoring health, through prolonging life and

---

[18] On the concept, see Csordas 1994; Bermúdez et al. 1998; Williams and Bendelow 1998; Lakoff and Johnson 1999; Komjathy 2005.

developing martial prowess, to cultivating energetic awareness and reaching mystical communion. They can achieve any of these, because Qigong is basically a series of efficacious systems that leads people to encounter a new way of experiencing and seeing the body, to have personal experiences with body-based transformations, and to discover the previously unknown ontological layer of *qi*. It is a way to put people back into their bodies and change the way they understand themselves in the world.

As Qigong spreads in American and other Western societies, it by necessity undergoes cultural adaptation. It reconstructs the history and concepts of Daoism in new ways, using perennial philosophy and New Age visions.

Created as an intentional secularization and medicalization of religious-based practices, Qigong is absorbed back into Daoist practice both in China and overseas and contributes to its formation in the 21st century. Just as the spread of Daoist teachings and practices into Western cultures leads to a new dimension of the religion, so the growth of the Qigong movement is in the process of leading to a reinterpretation of the religion. It is not what it used to be, and we do not know what it will be like. Studying Qigong in America is fascinating as it shows religion in the making and cultural interchange at its rawest front.

Bibliography

Abramson, John. 2004. *Overdo$ed America: The Broken Promise of American Medicine*. New York: HarperCollins.

Anderson, Poul. 1989. "A Visit to Hua Shan." *Cahiers d'Extreme-Asie* 5: 349-54.

Barnard, William. 2001. "Diving into the Depths: Reflections on Psychology as Religion." In *Religion and Psychology: Mapping the Terrain*, edited by Diane Jonte-Pace and William B. Parsons, 297-318. London and New York: Routledge.

Belamide, Paulino. 2000. "Taoism and Healing in North America: The Healing Tao of Mantak Chia." *International Review of Chinese Religion and Philosophy* 5: 245-89.

Bermúdez, José Luis, Anthony Marcel, and Naomi Eilan, eds. 1998. *The Body and the Self*. Cambridge, Mass.L: MIT Press.

Blofeld, John. 1973. *The Secret and the Sublime: Taoist Mysteries and Magic.* New York: Dutton.

Chang, Stephen T. 1978. *The Book of Internal Exercises.* San Francisco: Strawberry Hill Press.

Chen Hui-xian, with Holly Ann Alswel. 1995. *Finding Our Way Back Home: Soaring Crane Qigong II.* Portland, Ore.

_____. 1996. *Advanced Qigong.* Edited by Phyllis Lefohn. Portland, Ore.

Chen, Nancy N. 2003. *Breathing Spaces: Qigong, Psychiatry, and Healing in China.* New York: Columbia University Press.

Chia, Mantak. 1983. *Awaken Healing Energy through the Tao.* Introduced by Michael Winn. New York: Aurora Books.

_____. 1985. *Taoist Ways to Transform Stress into Vitality.* Huntington, NY: Healing Tao Books.

_____. 1986. *Iron Shirt Chi Kung I.* Huntington, NY: Healing Tao Books.

_____. 1993. *Awaken Healing Light of the Tao.* Huntington, NY: Healing Tao Books.

Cohen, Kenneth S. 1997. *The Way of Qigong: The Art and Science of Chinese Energy Healing.* New York: Ballantine Books.

_____. 2002a. "B. P. Chan: A True Person of No Rank." *Qi: The Journal of Traditional Eastern Health and Fitness* 12.2: 28-33.

_____. 2002b. "Taiji Ruler: Legacy of the Sleeping Immortal." Unpublished paper.

Csordas, Thomas J., ed. 1994. *Embodiment and Experience: The Existential Ground of Culture and Self.* Cambridge: Cambridge University Press.

Da Liu. 1972. *T'ai Chi Ch'uan and I Ching.* New York: Harper and Row.

_____. 1974. *Taoist Health Exercise Book.* New York: Paragon House.

_____. 1978. *The Tao of Health and Longevity.* Rev. ed. New York: Paragon House.

_____. 1979. *The Tao and Chinese Culture.* New York: Schocken Books.

Deng Ming-dao. 1993. *Chronicles of Tao: The Secret Life of a Taoist Master.* San Francisco: HarperSanFrancisco.

Ding Huang. 2000. "The Study of Daoism in China Today." In *Daoism Handbook*, edited by Livia Kohn, 765-91. Leiden: Brill.

Douglas, Bill. 2002. *The Complete Idiot's Guide to T'ai Chi and Qigong.* New York: Alpha Books.

Ferraro, Dominique. 2000. *Qigong for Women: Low-impact Exercises for Enhancing Energy and Toning the Body.* Rochester, VT: Healing Arts Press.

Garripoli, Garri (Francesco). 1999. *Qigong: Essence of the Healing Dance.* Deerfield Beach, FL: Health Communications, Inc.

Hanegraaff, Wouter J. 1998. *New Age Religion and Western Culture: Esotericism in the Mirror of Secular Thought.* Albany: State University of New York Press.

Happold, F. C. 1970. *Mysticism: A Study and an Anthology.* Baltimore: Penguin.

Huxley, Aldous. 1946. *The Perennial Philosophy.* New York and London: Harper & Brothers.

Iwamura, Jane. 2000. "The Oriental Monk in America Popular Culture." In *Religion and Popular Culture in America*, edited by Bruce David Forbes and Jeffrey H. Mahan. Berkeley: University of California Press.

Jahnke, Roger. 1999. *The Healer Within: Using Traditional Chinese Techniques to Release Your Body's Own Medicine.* San Francisco: HarperSanFrancisco.

_____. 2002. *The Healing Promise of Qi: Creating Extraordinary Wellness through Qigong and Tai Chi.* Columbus, Ohio: McGraw-Hill.

_____. 2005. "Varieties of Qigong." http://www.nqa.org/articles/varitiesofqigong.pdf. Accessed on 6/15/05.

Johnson, Jerry Alan. 2000. *Chinese Medical Qigong Therapy: A Comprehensive Clinical Text.* Pacific Grove, Calif.: International Institute of Medical Qigong.

Johnson, Larry. 1998. *18 Buddha Hands Qigong.* Crestone, Col.: White Elephant Monastery.

_____. 2001. *Strategies: Taoist Chi Kung—Level 1*. Crestone, Col.: White Elephant Monastery.

_____. 2002. *Strategies: Taoist Chi Kung—Levels 2 and 3*. Crestone, Col.: White Elephant Monastery.

Johnson, Yanling Lee. 2001. *A Woman's Qigong Guide: Empowerment through Movement, Diet, and Herbs*. Boston, Mass.: Yang's Martial Arts Association (YMAA) Publication Center.

Kirkland, Russell. 1997. "The Taoism of the Western Imagination and the Taoism of China: De-colonizing the Exotic Teachings of the East." www.arches.uga.edu/~kirkland/rk/pdf/pubs/pres/TENN97.pdf. Accessed on 6/15/05.

_____. 2004. *Taoism: The Enduring Tradition*. New York: Routledge.

Kleinman, Arthur. 1980. *Patients and Healers in the Context of Culture*. Berkeley: University of California Press.

Kohn, Livia, ed. 2000. *Daoism Handbook*. Leiden: Brill.

_____. 2001. *Daoism and Chinese Culture*. Cambridge, Mass.: Three Pines Press.

_____. 2004. *Cosmos and Community: The Ethnical Dimension of Daoism*. Cambridge, Mass.: Three Pines Press.

_____. 2005. *Health and Long Life: The Chinese Way*. Cambridge, Mass.: Three Pines Press.

_____. forthcoming. *Chinese Healing Exercises*. Magdalena, NM: Three Pines Press.

Komjathy, Louis. 2003a. "Daoist Teachers in North America." www.daoistcenter.org/articles.html. Accessed on 6/15/05.

_____. 2003b. "Daoist Organizations in North America." www.daoistcenter.org/articles.html. Accessed on 6/15/05.

_____. 2004. "Tracing the Contours of Daoism in North America." *Nova Religio* 8.2: 5-27.

_____. 2005. "Cultivating Perfection: Mysticism and Self-transformation in Early Quanzhen Daoism." Ph.D. diss., Boston University.

_____. forthcoming. "Mapping the Daoist Body: The Neijing tu and the Daoist Internal Landscape." *Journal of Chinese Religions* 34 (2006).

LaFargue, Michael, and Julian Pas. 1998. "On Translating the *Tao-te-ching*." In *Lao-tzu and the Tao-te-ching*, edited by Livia Kohn and Michael LaFargue, 277-302. Albany: State University of New York Press.

Lakoff, George, and Mark Johnson. 1999. *Philosophy in the Flesh: The Embodied Mind and Its Challenge to Western Thought*. New York: Basic Books.

Lau, Kimberly. 2000. *New Age Capitalism: Making Money East of Eden*. Philadelphia: University of Pennsylvania Press.

Lewis, James R., and J. Gordon Melton, eds. 1992. *Perspectives on the New Age*. Albany: State University of New York Press.

Liang, Shou-yu, and Wen-ching Wu. 1997. *Qigong Empowerment: A Guide to Medical, Taoist, Buddhist, Wushu Energy Cultivation*. East Providence, RI: The Way of the Dragon Publishing.

Liang, T. T. 1977. *T'ai Chi Ch'uan for Health and Self-defense*. New York: Vintage.

Liu, Yuzeng. 1999. *Wudang Qigong: China's Wudang Mountain Daoist Breath Exercises*. Translated by Liu Yuzeng and Terri Morgan. Overland Park, Kansas: International Wudang Internal Martial Arts.

Lu, K'uan-yü 1970. *Taoist Yoga: Alchemy and Immortality*. York Beach, Maine: Samuel Weiser.

Miller, James. 2003. *Daoism: A Short Introduction*. Oxford: Oneworld.

Min Zhiting 閔智亭. 1990. *Daojiao yifan* 道教儀範. Beijing: Zhongguo daojiao xueyuan bianyin.

Miura, Kunio. 1989. "The Revival of *Qi*: Qigong in Contemporary China." In *Taoist Meditation and Longevity Techniques*, edited by Livia Kohn, 331-62. Ann Arbor: Center for Chinese Studies, University of Michigan.

Morrison, Hedda. 1974. *Hua Shan: The Taoist Sacred Mountain in West China*. Hong Kong: Vetch and Lee.

Newton, Virginia. 2001. *Healing Energy: Master Zi Sheng Wang and Tibetan Buddhist Qigong*. San Francisco: China Books and Periodicals.

Olson, Stuart Alve. 1997. *Eight Brocades Seated Ch'i-kung*. Minneapolis, Minn.: Jade Forest Publishers.

_____. 2002a. *Qigong Teachings of a Taoist Immortal: The Eight Essential Exercises of Master Li Ching-yun.* Rochester, Vermont: Healing Arts Press.

_____. 2002b. *Steal My Art: The Life and Times of T'ai Chi Master T. T. Liang.* Berkeley: North Atlantic Press.

Palmer, David. 2005. *La fièvre du qigong. Guérison, religion et politique en Chine, 1949-1999.* Paris: Editions de l'Ecole des Hautes Etudes en Sciences Sociales.

_____. 2006. *Qigong Fever: Body, Knowledge and Power in Post-Mao China.* New York: Hurst & Co..

Reid, Daniel. 1998. *Harnessing the Power of the Universe: A Complete Guide to the Principles and Practice of Chi-gung.* Boston: Shambhala.

Roof, Wade Clark. 2001. *Spiritual Marketplace: Baby Boomers and the Remaking of American Religion.* Princeton: Princeton University Press.

Said, Edward. 1979. *Orientalism.* New York: Vintage Books.

Shih, T.K. 1989. *The Swimming Dragon: A Chinese Way to Fitness, Beautiful Skin, Weight Loss, and High Energy.* New York: Station Hill Press.

_____. 1994. *Qi Gong Therapy: The Chinese Art of Healing with Energy.* New York: Station Hill Press.

Siegler, Elijah. 2003. "The Dao of America: The History and Practice of American Daoism." Ph.D. diss., University of California, Santa Barbara.

Siou, Lily. 1973. *Ch'i Kung: The Art of Mastering the Unseen Life Force.* Honolulu: Lily Siou's School of The Six Chinese Arts.

_____. 1975. *Ch'i Kung: The Art of Mastering the Unseen Life Force.* Rutland, Vermont: Charles E. Tuttle Co.

Stone, Justin. 1996. *Tai Chi Chih! Joy Thru Movement.* Fort Yates, ND: Good Karma Publishing.

Towler, Solala. 1996. *A Gathering of Cranes: Bringing the Tao to the West.* Eugene, Ore.: Abode of the Eternal Tao.

_____. 1998. *Embarking on the Way: A Guide to Western Taoism.* Eugene, Ore.: Abode of the Eternal Tao.

Unschuld, Paul. 1985. *Medicine in China: A History of Ideas*. Berkeley: University of California Press.

Wessinger, Catherine. 2000. *How the Millennium Comes Violently: From Jonestown to Heaven's Gate*. New York and London: Seven Bridges Press.

Williams, Simon J. and Gillian Bendelow. 1998. *The Lived Body: Sociological Themes, Embodied Issues*. London and New York: Routledge.

Yang Jwing-ming. 1985. *Chi Kung—Health and Martial Arts*. Jamaica Plain, Mass.: Yang's Martial Arts Association Publication Center.

_____. 1988. *The Eight Pieces of Brocade*. Jamaica Plain, Mass.: Yang's Martial Arts Association Publication Center.

_____. 1989a. *The Root of Chinese Chi Kung: The Secrets of Chi Kung Training*. Jamaica Plain, Mass.: Yang's Martial Arts Association Publication Center.

_____. 1989b. *Muscle/Tendon Changing and Marrow/Brain Washing Chi Kung: The Secret of Youth*. Jamaica Plain, Mass.: Yang's Martial Arts Association Publication Center.

_____. 2003. *Qigong Meditation: Embryonic Breathing*. Jamaica Plain, Mass.: Yang's Martial Arts Association Publication Center.

Index